Cardiothoracic Surgical Nursing

Carl Margereson
MSc BSc(Hons) DipN(Lond) RGN RMN
Senior Lecturer
Faculty of Health & Human Sciences
Thames Valley University

Jillian Riley
MSc BA(Hons) RGN RM
Senior Lecturer
Faculty of Health & Human Sciences
Thames Valley University
Royal Brompton Hospital, London

Blackwell
Science

Editorial offices:
Blackwell Science Ltd, 9600 Garsington Road,
Oxford OX4 2DQ, UK
  Tel: +44 (0)1865 776868
Blackwell Publishing Inc., 350 Main Street,
Malden, MA 02148-5020, USA
  Tel: +1 781 388 8250
Blackwell Science Asia Pty Ltd, 550 Swanston
Street, Carlton, Victoria 3053, Australia
  Tel: +61 (0)3 8359 1011

First published 2003

Library of Congress
Cataloging-in-Publication Data
Margereson, Carl.
   Cardiothoracic surgical nursing: current trends
in adult care/Carl Margereson, Jillian Riley. – 1st
ed.
      p. ; cm.
Includes bibliographical references and index.
   ISBN 0-632-05904-4 (pbk. : alk. paper)
1. Chest – Surgery – Nursing.
2. Heart – Surgery – Nursing.
   [DNLM: 1. Perioperative Nursing – trends.
2. Thoracic Surgical Procedures – nursing.
3. Cardiovascular Diseases – nursing.
4. Nurse's Role.   5. Patient Education.
6. Respiratory Tract Diseases – nursing.
WY 161 M328c 2003]

   RD536.M275 2003
   617.5′4059 – dc21

                                    2003010441

ISBN 0-632-05904-4

A catalogue record for this title is available
from the British Library

Set in 10/12pt Palatino
by DP Photosetting, Aylesbury, Bucks
Printed and bound in Great Britain using
acid-free paper by TJ International Ltd,
Padstow, Cornwall

For further information on
Blackwell Publishing, visit our website:
www.blackwellpublishing.com

Contents

Foreword

I was both delighted and honoured when asked by Carl and Jill to write the foreword to this excellent nursing book. Having worked with them in varying capacities over the past six years, I have long appreciated their knowledge, understanding and expertise within this specialist field of patient care. When any author sets out to write, the most important tool for the task is credibility. It is upon this foundation that the book is written, with both authors having shaped nursing practice for many years through their teaching and encouragement of post registration nurses who accessed ENB 249 and 254 courses. Both authors remain firmly in touch with the contemporary issues that influence nursing within a modern NHS, and are respected for their ongoing support of the clinical team. A vital contribution of health care educators and their ability to help shape patient care in the twenty-first century.

The book itself is written with this in mind. It is not a reflective dialogue of the many changes and challenges that the nursing profession have had to meet head on over the past two decades. It is more a recognition of where the profession and cardiothoracic surgical nursing are at, and how they need to continue to develop. It reflects current socio-political and professional thinking, in mapping the patient journey from early symptoms, hospitalisation through to returning home. It successfully enables the reader to appreciate the size of the challenge from an epidemiological perspective; deepens their understanding of physiological and pathophysiological principles; maps the patient journey in the peri-operative period, through the experience of surgery to post-operative recovery and reha-bilitation. This book is not a snapshot of cardiothoracic surgical patient care, but more a considered and reflective account that is based on understanding and intuition of how nurses can meet the challenges of patients and their families' needs.

It is written with the post-registration student in mind, supporting many of the excellent undergraduate specialist cardiothoracic pathways that shape both thinking and practice. To this end it will be an invaluable test, giving wide coverage of the essential areas of knowledge and expertise that the cardiothoracic surgical nurse needs to develop. It reflects the authors' passion for the subject, their compassion for the patient and their commitment to the profession. Enjoy the journey.

Dr Ian Bullock
Head of Education and Training
Royal Brompton and Harefield NHS Trust

Preface

Cardiothoracic surgical nursing has undergone immense change over the past decade, owing in part to professional, economic and societal changes. The profile of patients undergoing cardiothoracic surgery has also changed as cardiothoracic surgery is performed upon the more elderly, the high-risk or those with co-morbidity. Although previously considered at too high a risk for surgery, improved surgical techniques, pharmacology and pre- and post-operative care have resulted in a successful outcome for many patients and a return to an improved quality of life.

The specialisation of cardiothoracic nursing has developed to meet the challenge of the above changes. However, at this time, there is ongoing debate regarding evolving roles, blurring of professional boundaries, generic practitioners and a multi-skilled workforce. Cardiothoracic nurses must remain focused upon their unique contribution to patient outcome, and this text explores some of these important issues. Yet as these developments continue, nursing research and education must also keep up the pace. For example, nursing interventions such as new models for patient education or rehabilitation must develop from an evidence base.

This text has posed a challenge to the authors. Even during its writing, practices have changed. One such change resulted from the patient choice initiative, which in itself provides the cardiothoracic surgical nurse with many more challenges and opportunities. We hope that this will be a useful text for nurses working in this exciting field and that it may contribute in some way to the development of innovative and creative cardiothoracic nursing practice.

Carl Margereson and Jillian Riley

Acknowledgements

There are so many people to thank, including our many colleagues and friends who have contributed to the development of this book both wittingly and unwittingly. However, first of all our heartfelt thanks must go to all the patients over the years, who have placed themselves in our care and who have been instrumental in helping us to hone our nursing skills, not only as practitioners but also as educators. We would also like to acknowledge the help of our colleagues at Thames Valley University and Royal Brompton Hospital who have shared the journey with us. Special thanks must go to Dr Ian Bullock and senior nurses Linda Hart and Elizabeth Allibone for reviewing sections of the book.

We must also thank Karen Philipson and Dr Hilary Adams who generously gave their time to read early drafts of the manuscript. Over the years we have had the pleasure of teaching so many nurses who have completed our cardiothoracic courses. This short book was written with them in mind and we hope it serves as a useful text for others.

1

The Development of Cardiothoracic Surgical Nursing

Cardiothoracic surgical nursing is currently undergoing immense change. This has been assisted by several factors: the recent government papers such as the National Service Frameworks (DoH 2000a) and the NHS Plan (DoH 2000b), the shift in care towards greater patient acuity in hospital and more specialist care in the community, improved technology and drug therapy, and the growing number of older people undergoing major surgery. There have also been major professional, economic and societal changes that have impacted not only upon the management of the patient journey but also upon patient expectations.

Cardiothoracic surgery has developed tremendously over the past years. It was following the removal of bullets from the chest, particularly during World War II, that the early pioneers of surgery realised that the heart could be successfully manipulated during surgery (Cooley & Frazier 2000). This led to the beginnings of cardiac surgery, although upon a closed heart. The Vineberg operation was used to implant the internal mammary artery directly into the left ventricle, and successfully relieved angina (Thomas 2000). However, it was not until the early 1950s and the development of the cardiopulmonary bypass circuit, that open-heart surgery could develop towards that known today. Around this same time, major developments in positive pressure ventilation improved the post-operative management of patients and contributed to successful outcomes. The first coronary artery bypass surgery was performed in 1964 (Cooley & Frazier 2000) and since then surgery for revascularisation has developed further. Resulting from advances in both technology and pharmacology, current work surrounds beating heart, minimally invasive and endoscopic cardiac surgery.

There have been similar developments in the treatment of valvular heart disease, where the dilation of stenosed valves with the finger and mechanical dilators has led to the use of balloons inserted percutaneously for the same purpose. Valve replacement with mechanical valves enabled both the stenosed and regurgitant valve to be corrected. From the early ball and cage device, tissue valves such as homograft valves are now used in increasing numbers.

Thoracic surgery has also developed over the past 50 years, largely owing to improvement in anaesthetic techniques and post-operative ventilatory support.

1

Since the 1980s, progress has included developments in both lung and heart transplantation with improved techniques for tracheal resection and reconstruction. The use of video-assisted techniques of thoracic surgery and lung volume reduction for emphysema continues to gather momentum. An important factor, which will dictate how thoracic surgery evolves over the next decade, is cancer research. It is predicted that staging will be enhanced by monoclonal antibodies and new technology and that more lung-sparing techniques will be carried out with expansion of pre-operative and post-operative adjuvant treatment programmes (Faber 1993).

Thoracic surgical procedures range from those which are relatively straightforward to those where risk is considerable. The profile of patients coming forward for surgery varies enormously, from the young, fit male requiring pleurodesis, to the high-risk patient who requires major reconstructive surgery perhaps because of malignancy. This great range poses a real challenge to the cardiothoracic nurse as health needs vary greatly between individuals and across different patient groups, with outcome often difficult to predict.

Specialisation in medicine and surgery has led to many scientific advances, and expert practice has evolved as a result of specialisation in surgery. This has been mirrored in nursing, where practitioners have focused on either cardiac or thoracic care in terms of career development. The pernicious effects of sub-specialisation have been commented upon, and it is argued that there is danger of the speciality as an entity being diminished (Anderson 1999). Such a trend could also contribute to some areas being underfunded in terms of research and training where 'cutting edge' initiatives receive the lion's share of resources, leaving other areas struggling. If funding is poor for medical research and education in some of the less glamorous areas of cardiothoracic work, then funding for nursing is likely to be even worse.

Given the scale of respiratory disease in the UK today it is unfortunate that the government does not appear to see this as a priority, as at the time of writing there is still no national service framework for respiratory illness. Partridge (2002) argues that, in the management of lung cancer, the same surgeons who are being pressured to deliver results in coronary artery bypass surgery are also being asked to provide prompt surgery for lung cancer. Yet with 40,000 new cases of lung cancer in the UK each year, only 10% of patients have lung resections compared with 24% in Holland (Damhuis & Schutte 1996) and 25% in the USA (Fry & Menck 1996). With the current pattern of pulmonary morbidity there will be an increasing need for thoracic surgeons and cardiothoracic nurses for quite some time to come.

With all the developments in cardiothoracic surgery, many patients previously considered too high a risk for surgery, are now operated upon and the skills of the whole team have had to grow to accommodate these changes. For some cardiothoracic surgical nurses this has resulted in the development of acute care skills and learning new techniques to manage and support the post-operative course. For the patient, these advances have led to less risk of complications, a shorter hospital stay and a quicker return to an active life (Dunstan & Riddle 1977). Yet this shorter stay has decreased the contact time of the hospital nurse with the patient. It emphasises the need to alter models of care delivery while raising the importance of bridging the hospital–community interface through schemes such as 'Hospital at home' and liaison services (Penque *et al.* 1999; Brennan *et al.* 2001). Performing surgery on the elderly or on those with co-morbidity also has a huge social impact and developments in social care and health care must continue in parallel. Operating on the sick or elderly, only to have them remain in hospital with the increased likelihood of developing hospital-acquired complications, would appear to be counterproductive.

Another major development over the past decade has been in the pre-operative assessment and preparation for surgery, and this is likely to continue as nurses develop a more proactive, specialist role in coordinating the patient journey. Possibly started from an interest in rehabilitation and fuelled by the National Service Framework for coronary heart disease (DoH 2000a) and the NHS modernisation plan (DoH 2000b), the concepts of pre-operative assessment, fitness for surgery and the expert patient have developed. The cardiothoracic surgical nurse has consequently developed knowledge and skills in health promotion, secondary prevention and rehabilitation (Latter *et al.* 1992). Cardiothoracic surgery is frequently associated with a position of ill health, which may be influenced favourably by the surgery itself. This means that the cardiothoracic surgical nurse, while caring for the individual when sick, is in a position to offer health promotion advice as well and to assist the patient to reach their full health potential.

The nursing profession has also driven several of these changes, initiating nursing roles and alternative models of health care. The *Scope of Professional Practice* (UKCC 1992) may have given rise to the dawn of many of these roles. It enabled individual nurses to take responsibility for their actions and the expansion of their services. It emphasised professional accountability in deciding the boundaries of each individual nurse's responsibility and enabled roles such as the nurse anaesthetist or surgeon's assistant to become established. These nurses, through embodying the focus of nursing, accompany surgeons on ward rounds and undertake physical assessments and thus contribute towards the whole assessment process. More recently there has been the development of independent roles such as the nurse consultant (Manley 1997), an expert practitioner in nursing a specific patient group. Possibilities for their role in the care of the patient undergoing cardiothoracic surgery are therefore clear: assisting the provision of seamless care from the pre-admission preparation to returning home, providing an expert outreach service, managing ventilator or inotropic weaning are a few examples.

Yet the care of the cardiothoracic surgical patient requires teamwork from both within and without the hospital setting. Understanding the contribution that each profession makes to the team is not straightforward. Learning together and what has come to be referred to as interprofessional learning, may enhance clinical effectiveness through increased understanding of each professions role (DoH 1997; Rolls *et al.* 2002). An early example of this in the UK is in the teaching of advanced life support skills. This approach has proved successful in developing the emergency team for cardiac arrest (Nolan & Mitchell 1999; Bullock 2000). It serves to bring the professions together and develop the necessary knowledge and skills while demonstrating the unique contribution that each profession has to patient care and outcome. However, there has also been much recent discussion upon flexible multi-professional teamwork and cross-boundary working. These developments should be regarded cautiously for their implications for the future of the nursing profession.

Education will continue to be important in the development of the cardio-thoracic surgical nurse. Pre-registration courses prepare nurses to work in a variety of care settings, yet specialist care requires further development of this knowledge and skills, and cardiothoracic courses are now offered at degree level. Within such specialist education, research must also be given a greater emphasis as nurses develop the evidence for care and evaluate new practices. Nursing therefore has to plan a framework for this career development that encourages the development of the cardiothoracic surgical nurse from post-registration towards doctorate level and beyond (Riley *et al.* 2003). Figure 1.1 outlines a possible framework.

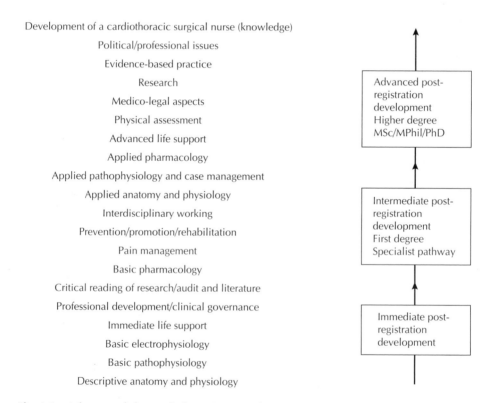

Fig. 1.1   A framework for cardiothoracic surgical nursing.

We should also want our profession to provide for the education of those who follow. This was reflected in the grading system for nurses, making explicit their role as a teacher, and is an important component of the nurse consultant role (Manley 1997). The continued development of cardiothoracic surgical nursing requires expertise in enabling others to learn so that the same high standards of care delivered by us to our patients can be preserved and developed further in those that follow. Thus, both the science and art of nursing may be taught and preserved. Utilising examples of clinical nursing and acting as role models may be an effective way to achieve this, and the pre-admission clinic provides an excellent forum for learning, enabling the nurse to develop skills in both the interpretation of physiological data, psychological assessment, communication and patient education.

Evidence-based health care is also gaining popularity. It is increasingly important that nursing interventions are derived from a research base and able to withstand strict scrutiny. Purchasers of health care, patients and their families both expect and deserve the best care, and nursing actions should be evaluated and developed. So nurses must incorporate nursing research into their practice, appraising research, implementing findings and developing new studies. Although the current climate suggests that randomised controlled trials are the gold standard for research, such trials may not be the most appropriate method to study the individual response to treatment. Nursing research should continue to adopt a multiple paradigm approach.

Cardiothoracic surgery has undergone major developments over the past 80 years, which have moved the service forward in a way that previously was only dreamt about. Yet the provision of care continues to require a careful balance of both the art and science of nursing. By ensuring this balance, we can continue to provide skilful, decisive and compassionate care.

References

Anderson, R.P. (1999) Thoracic surgery at century's end. *Annals of Thoracic Surgery* **67**: 897–902.

Brennan, P., Moore, S., Bkornsdottir, G., Jones, J., Visovsky, C. & Rogers., M. (2001) Heartcare: an internet based information and support system for patient home recovery after coronary artery bypass grafting surgery. *Journal of Advanced Nursing* **35**(5): 699–708.

Bullock, I. (2000) Skill acquisition in resuscitation. *Resuscitation* **45**: 139–43.

Cooley, D. & Frazier, O. (2000) The past 50 years of cardiovascular surgery. *Circulation* **102**(20): 87–93.

Damhuis, R.A. & Schutte, P.R. (1996) Resection rates and postoperative mortality in 7,899 patients with lung cancer. *European Respiratory Journal* **9**: 7–10.

DoH (Department of Health) (1997) *The New NHS: Modern, Dependable*. The Stationery Office, London.

DoH (Department of Health) (2000a) *The National Service Framework for Coronary Heart Disease*. The Stationery Office, London.

DoH (Department of Health) (2000b) *The NHS Plan: A Plan for Investment, A Plan for Reform*. The Stationery Office, London.

Dunstan, J. & Riddle, M. (1997) Rapid recovery management: the effects on the patient who has undergone heart surgery. *Heart and Lung* **26**(4): 289–98.

Faber, P.L. (1993) General thoracic surgery in the year 2010. *Annals of Thoracic Surgery* **55**: 1326–31.

Fry, W.A. & Menck, H.R. (1996) The national cancer data base report on lung cancer. *Cancer* **77**: 1947–55.

Latter, S., MacCleod-Clark, J., Wilson-Barnett, J. & Maben, J. (1992) Health education in nursing: perceptions of practice in acute settings. *Journal of Advanced Nursing* **17**(2): 164–72.

Manley, K. (1997) A conceptual framework for advanced practice: an action research project operationalising and advanced practitioner/consultant nurse role. *Journal of Clinical Nursing* **6**(3): 179–90.

Nolan, J. & Mitchell, S. (1999) The advanced life support course and requirements of the Royal Colleges. *Resuscitation* **41**: 211.

Partridge, M.R. (2002) Thoracic surgery in a crisis: New report outlines dire shortage of thoracic surgeons. *British Medical Journal* **324**(7334): 376–7.

Penque, S., Petersen, B., Arom, K., Ratner, E. & Halm, M. (1999) Early discharge with home health care in the coronary artery bypass patient. *Dimensions of Critical Care Nursing* **18**(6): 40–48.

Riley, J., Bullock, I., West, S. & Shuldham, C. (2003) Practical application of educational rhetoric: a pathway to expert cardiac nursing practice?

Rolls, L., Davis, E. & Coupland, K. (2002) Improving serious mental illness through interprofessional education. *Journal of Psychiatric and Mental Health Nursing* **9**(3): 317–24.

Thomas, J. (2000) The Vineberg legacy: internal mammary artery implantation from inception to obsolescence. *Texas Heart Institute Journal* **27**(1): 80–81.

UKCC (United Kingdom Central Council for Nursing, Midwifery and Health Visiting) (1992) *The Scope of Professional Practice*. UKCC, London.

Epidemiology of Cardiac and Respiratory Diseases

In the nineteenth century, life expectancy was only around 40 years, but today it has almost doubled at 74 years for men and 78 years for women. Over the past 100 years there have been major changes in the causes of death in developed countries, with circulatory disease and cancer taking over from infectious diseases. In poorer countries, however, communicable diseases remain the major cause of death. Worldwide, cardiovascular diseases are the most common cause of death and a substantial source of chronic disability and health care costs. Primary care consultations are far greater for respiratory problems than any other disease group and this has been increasing over the past 15 years. However, respiratory problems are still grossly under-recognised. The British Lung Foundation (1996) suggests that 50 years ago no one would have predicted the prevalence of respiratory disease both nationally and worldwide.

Cardiac disease

In the UK there has been a decline in the death rate from coronary heart disease (CHD) for adults under the age of 75 years by 31% over the past ten years but unfortunately the rate is still among the highest in the world. In the UK, cardio-vascular disease accounts for over 235 000 deaths a year, mainly CHD and stroke. CHD is the most common cause of death in the UK, with 125 000 deaths a year accounting for 1 in 4 deaths in men (Fig. 2.1(a)) and 1 in 6 in women (Fig. 2.1(b)). CHD is responsible for 24% of premature deaths in men and 14% in women. There are 149 000 heart attacks each year in men of all ages and about 125 000 each year in women, an approximate fatality rate of 50%, with 25–30% dying before reaching

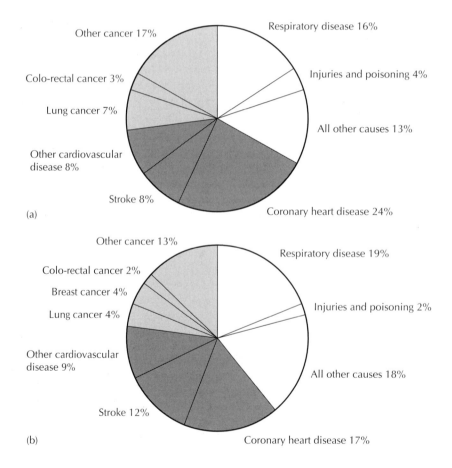

Fig. 2.1   Deaths by cause, 2000, UK. (a) Men. (b) Women. From Petersen & Rayner (2002), with permission.

hospital. In the UK, 1.1 million men and 1 million women have had angina. There is little data on heart failure but the crude incidence rate is 140 per 100 000 annually for men and 120 per 100 000 for women, with 33 000 and 30 000 new cases, respectively, in the UK (Petersen & Rayner 2002).

In economic terms, CHD costs the UK health service about £1.6 billion a year, with hospital care accounting for 55% of the cost. Only a very modest amount of this (1%), however, is spent on the prevention of CHD. In total, with loss of income, CHD cost the UK more than £8.5 billion in 1996 (Petersen & Rayner 2002). Health service expenditure includes about 28 000 angioplasties and just under 28 000 coronary bypass operations each year, although rates vary between National Health Service districts.

Although the incidence of valvular heart disease in the UK has reduced over the past 50 years, it is still responsible for significant morbidity. This decline has been led by the reduction in rheumatic heart disease seen throughout the western world (Julian *et al.* 1996). However, with the global movement of populations this pattern appears to be changing and the current re-emergence of rheumatic heart disease in the UK may yet lead to an increase in the number of people developing mitral valve disease. Interestingly, although this has led to a reduction in the number of people with mitral valve disease, the increased longevity of life enjoyed by many has led to a corresponding increase in the number of people presenting with stenosis of the aortic valve. Although the process of aortic valve stenosis is now thought to be inflammatory rather than degenerative, symptoms are more likely to occur in those aged between 70 and 80 years (Otto 2002). In a subset of these, surgical replacement will be required.

The number of adults with congenital heart disease is also increasing and this has been influenced by improvements in management during childhood. Surgical techniques and pharmacological therapy have developed, while there has been some improvement noted in socio-economic situations. People with complex heart defects are increasingly living into adulthood where they may develop further problems with their congenital heart defect or even acquired heart disease. This will add to the complexity of cardiothoracic surgical nursing over the next few decades.

Respiratory disease

In a recent publication, statistical data was for the first time, made available regarding the total impact of respiratory disease in the UK (British Thoracic Society 2001). This data shows that respiratory disease now kills more people than CHD, and in 1999 was responsible for 153 000 deaths. Since 1968, the death rate from respiratory disease has decreased by 31% while death rates from CHD have fallen by around 53%. The total cost to the NHS of all respiratory diseases was over £2.5 billion in 2000. Although respiratory problems are the largest single cause of certified absence from work in both men and women, with 7% of adults reporting long-term respiratory illness, not all require surgical intervention. In 1999/2000 there were 10 500 operations for respiratory disease with 40% (4288) being for the treatment of lung cancer (British Thoracic Society 2001).

Lung cancer

Lung cancer accounts for 20% of all cancers and is responsible for 24% of all cancer deaths in the UK (Doll & Peto 1996). Overwhelming evidence has been available for some time to show that smoking is a major cause of lung cancer, but with many people still smoking, physicians and surgeons are likely to be busy for some time yet, with 40 000 new cases diagnosed each year.

Resection of a tumour offers the best chance of a cure and this is an option mainly for patients with stage I or II non-small-cell lung cancer, where 30% may be responsive (Morgan 1996). More effective staging procedures have led to a fall in the number of patients undergoing unnecessary thoracotomy, but the five-year survival rate is still only 35–40%. The extent of the procedure will depend on many factors not least the patient's general condition but may include removal of a whole lung (mortality 8%), lobe (mortality <2%), segment or wedge (mortality 0.5%). Recent studies have shown that specialist management is associated with better outcomes than management by non-specialists, and patients should have access to tertiary services for thoracic surgery (DoH 1998).

Advanced age need not preclude surgical intervention for lung cancer and in appropriately selected patients mortality rates are similar to those seen in younger patients (Pagni *et al*. 1998; Hanagiri *et al*. 1999). However, pneumonectomy carries significantly higher risk for elderly patients. Further randomised controlled data is needed regarding induction chemotherapy in stage II or IIIA disease and the comparative role of radiotherapy in patients with poor respiratory function or with chest wall involvement (Edwards & Waller 2001).

Chronic obstructive pulmonary disease

Chronic obstructive pulmonary disease (COPD) is very common in the UK, with consultation rates estimated to be four times greater than those for angina (British Thoracic Society 1997). In general practice the consultation rates per 10 000 population rise from 417 at age 45–64, to 886 at age 65–74 and 1032 at age 75–84. Only 1 in 4 cases are recognised and the quality of life of people with COPD is among the worse of all chronic illness groups. Two main disorders fall under this heading: chronic bronchitis and emphysema. Smoking is the major cause of both diseases. A small subgroup of patients with emphysema have a deficiency of α_1 anti-trypsin.

Treatment of COPD consists mainly of smoking cessation and drug therapy with anticholinergics (ipratropium bromide) and β_2 agonists (salbutamol). Antibiotics are required for secondary infection. Steroids may be prescribed, although generally, results are disappointing. Domiciliary oxygen may be required for patients with chronic respiratory failure. As the disease progresses, for selected patients surgery may be considered including bullectomy, lung volume reduction and single lung transplantation.

Bronchiectasis

Bronchiectasis is a disorder of the respiratory tract where damage to the large airways results in abnormal dilation with poor clearance and pooling of mucus

(Cole 1995). This damage may occur as a result of earlier pathology such as whooping cough, pneumonia and measles. Although bronchiectasis may be initiated in childhood, as a rule problems do not manifest until adulthood when individuals are prone to chronic lower respiratory tract infections (Wilson *et al.* 1997). Treatment is usually medical, with intensive postural drainage. Recurrent infections with pneumonia despite maximum therapy may necessitate surgical resection of affected lung portions.

Interstitial lung disease

Interstitial lung disease (ILD) involves inflammation of the alveolar walls and adjacent spaces and includes around 130 different disorders, some of which may progress to a fibrosing stage eventually causing respiratory failure. Interstitial lung diseases are viewed as a diverse group of disorders classified together because of common clinical, radiographic, physiological and pathological features (Bouros *et al.* 1997). Most patients present with insidious onset of exertional breathlessness and diffuse alveolar or interstitial pattern on chest radiography. Cryptogenic (idiopathic) fibrosing alveolitis (CFA) is an ILD with the worst prognosis and the median survival is five years with only 25% of patients obtaining objective improvement to corticosteroid therapy (Turner-Warwick *et al.* 1980; du Bois 1990). There is also a greater risk of patients with CFA developing lung cancer.

For many patients with ILD the major physiological features will be breathlessness on exertion due to oxygen desaturation during exercise, chronic dry cough, eventual hypoxaemia and hypercapnia and finally respiratory and heart failure (Fulmer 1982). The pulmonary changes in ILD result in a restrictive ventilatory pattern. This is in contrast to the obstructive pattern seen in disorders such as COPD and asthma. A restrictive ventilatory pattern typically presents with:

- reduced lung volume and compliance
- minimal derangement of airflow
- impaired gas exchange
- pulmonary hypertension

Although the mainstay of treatment for many patients with ILD is pharmacological, often with powerful immunosuppressive agents, for some interstitial diseases (e.g. idiopathic pulmonary fibrosis) single lung transplantation may be possible for selected patients with end-stage disease (Sulica *et al.* 2001). Although early mortality is high (9–14%) in some groups, survival benefit has been demonstrated with transplantation in patients with idiopathic pulmonary fibrosis compared with medical treatment (Hosenpud *et al.* 1998) and improvements have been shown in lung volumes, exercise tolerance, gas exchange, pulmonary haemodynamics (Grossman *et al.* 1990; Bjortuft *et al.* 1996) and quality of life (Stavem *et al.* 2000). Unfortunately, despite increasing numbers presenting for transplantation there has not been a corresponding increase in available organs.

Other respiratory disorders

Examples of other disorders which may require thoracic surgical intervention include:

- Removal of benign tumours (5% of all lung tumours)
- Oesophageal carcinoma
- Removal of cysts (e.g. epithelial and emphysematous)
- Pneumothorax
- Pleural effusions (malignant/non malignant)
- Lung abscess
- Empyema thoracis
- Correction of pectus excavatum (funnel chest) and pectus carinatum (pigeon chest)

Epidemiology and risk factors

Epidemiology is an important science and epidemiologists have assumed a more dominant role in contemporary health care policy. It is epidemiology which measures how healthy and unhealthy we are at both national and local levels. The incidence and prevalence of various diseases can be determined, and by studying demographic changes, predictions and suggestions can be made about the course which effective health care policy should take. Epidemiological studies can identify patterns regarding the occurrence of individual diseases together with possible risk factors, which can be further tested in intervention studies where the impact on health of any risk modification is measured. Epidemiology is an intrinsic part of the public health movement.

Why is epidemiology important for surgical nurses caring for patients following cardiothoracic surgery? Health services are under ever increasing pressure, and with finite resources health spending needs to be a rational process based on sound epidemiological studies and valid assessment of need. Awareness of the wider issues of health care, particularly concerning resource allocation in cardiac and respiratory disease, is vital so that nurses can contribute to the ongoing debate in this area. Developing effective health care models where nurses have a more proactive role is not without resource implications, and appropriate evidence needs to be presented in an authoritative way.

Surgical nurses have an important role to play in health promotion, and findings from epidemiological studies can be useful here too. Knowledge of risk factors is necessary where assistance with lifestyle modification may be needed. An overview of risk factors is given later in this section. Although patients will need specific information about their surgical recovery, for example wound care and medication, other information regarding how to optimise health in general should be available and is often welcome. This is important not only for patients with cardiac disease but also for those undergoing thoracic surgery and indeed all patient groups that the nurse might encounter. Any health promotion, however, needs to be realistic as the goals will vary from patient to patient. Although group sessions are useful, they often need to be followed up with individual consultation.

Many might argue that with upcoming surgery, modification of lifestyle is the last thing on the patient's mind. However, in the pre-operative period, knowledge and skill deficits can be identified and these can be addressed subsequently in the post-operative period and following discharge. Periods of hospitalisation for surgery are shorter nowadays with more cases performed on a day-case basis. The nurse should not only be concerned with the period of hospitalisation but also ensure that health care delivery programmes in the surgical setting meet the health promotion needs of patients, if not during, then before and following hospitalisation.

Any attempt to assist in lifestyle modification must, however, be carried out with a sound knowledge of causation. Heart and lung disease are not simply caused by unhealthy diets, smoking and other risky behaviours. Both medical and social models of health need to be employed to understand causation and to develop effective intervention strategies. Knowledge of the many different factors involved in the development of disease will help to ensure that any health promotion role is carried out realistically and sensitively. We are deluged by the media with stories of various risks we are exposed to, and this often generates a great deal of confusion. The nurse should be a useful resource for the patient and be able to offer suggestions on how to promote health in the recovery period following surgery and beyond. Keeping abreast of all developments in this area is therefore crucial.

Risk factors

Many prospective epidemiological studies have been undertaken not only regarding the prevalence of heart disease but also to identify risk factors which predict to some degree the CHD mortality rate. Identified risk factors are important both for assessment of risk and as targets for interventions. Risk factors may be classified as follows (Grundy 1999):

■ Causal
■ Conditional
■ Predisposing

Causal risk factors

Major causal risk factors for CHD are cigarette smoking; high blood pressure; elevated LDL, low HDL cholesterol; high triglycerides; and high plasma glucose (Wilson *et al.* 1998). The importance of these risk factors was first highlighted by two important longitudinal studies: the British Regional Heart Study (Shaper *et al.* 1981) and the Framingham Study (Dawber 1980). It is assumed that if both the risk of the disease and the risk of death from all causes are reduced, then the factor is an independent causal risk factor.

Smoking

An important 40-year longitudinal study in the UK demonstrated conclusively the association between smoking and the development of a number of diseases, including heart disease and lung cancer (Doll *et al.* 1994). In patients with CHD, smoking is responsible for 20% of male deaths and 17% of female deaths, and yet 28% of men and 26% of women in the UK still smoke. Health behaviours are extremely complex and some of the cognitions responsible for behaviour are very resistant to modification. Cigarette smoking in adolescents is increasing, particularly among girls. About 9% of boys and 11% of girls aged 11–15 years are regular smokers. Although overall there has been a decline in smoking, rates vary across different age groups.

It is argued that half of all smokers will die of a smoking-related disease; half in middle age and half in old age, with a 1 in 4 risk of dying in middle age, so losing 20–25 years of a non-smoker's life expectancy (Peto *et al.* 1996). Passive smoking is now taken more seriously as far as it increases the risk of ischaemic heart disease and respiratory disease (Tunstall-Pedoe *et al.* 1995).

Cholesterol

Average levels of cholesterol in the UK are 5.5 mmol/l for men and over 5.6 mmol for women, although significant numbers have levels above 6.5 mmol/l (Lockhart *et al.* 2000). The strength of the relationship between cholesterol and CHD is greatest in younger people (Law *et al.* 1994). Ideal levels for total cholesterol should be 5 mmol/l and below, and less than 3 mmol/l for low-density lipoproteins (LDL). There is evidence to show that certain statins can reduce both risk and incidence of myocardial infarction (MI) (Evans & Rees 2002), although these should only be used in primary prevention of MI in high-risk patients in addition to other interventions such as exercise and dietary modification.

Plant sterols

There is evidence to suggest that plant sterols have a dose-dependent effect, lowering LDL cholesterol levels, while raising HDL (high-density lipoprotein) cholesterol. Sterols are similar to cholesterol but are not absorbed in the human gastrointestinal tract and also have the ability to inhibit the absorption of cholesterol. Various margarines have been marketed containing plant sterols but it is important to remember that these are still high in calories.

Polyunsaturated fatty acids and antioxidants

Increased intake of oily fish containing large amounts of n-3 polyunsaturated fatty acids (PUFAs) have been linked with a reduced incidence of CHD. And while there is support for the use of antioxidants in inhibiting the processes of atherosclerosis and thrombosis (Diaz *et al.* 1997), there is inadequate evidence from large randomised trials to support benefits from antioxidant supplementation (Tribble 1999). General advice should include consumption of a balanced diet with emphasis on antioxidant-rich fruit and vegetables and whole grains. Antioxidants may protect against free-radical-initiated damage and protect LDL cholesterol from oxidation. Similarly there are suggestions that antioxidants may have some effect on preventing pulmonary tissue damage, although work in this area is ongoing.

Flavonoids

There has been a great deal of attention in the popular press given to the protective effects of flavonoids. These are a large group of polyphenolic antioxidants that occur naturally in vegetables and fruits and in beverages such as tea and wine. Flavonoids in regularly consumed foods may reduce the risk of death from CHD in elderly men (Hertog 1993).

Alcohol

Patients often seek information about alcohol intake. The benefits of regular, light alcohol consumption for middle-aged men and women has been highlighted (DoH 1995). Abstainers have a greater burden of ill health than moderate drinkers, regardless of their previous drinking status. The protective effect of moderate alcohol consumption is related to (Criqui & Ringel 1994):

■ Increase in HDL
■ Reduction in plasma fibrinogen
■ Decreased platelet aggregation
■ Reduced triglycerides

The protective effect against CHD in moderate drinkers is lost rapidly if they stop drinking. Excessive alcohol intake will increase blood pressure, but regular consumption of moderate alcohol can reduce the build-up of fibrous plaque and reduce likelihood of a blood clot. Consumption of one alcoholic drink every one to two days appears to have a lower risk of myocardial infarction compared with either heavy alcohol or abstention (Mukamal *et al.* 2001).

Blood pressure

Raised blood pressure is a major risk factor for stroke and CHD, with 40% attributable to a systolic blood pressure of >140 mmHg (Marmot 1992). Blood pressure levels are high in the UK yet for each 5 mmHg reduction in blood pressure the risk of CHD is reduced by about 16%. The British Hypertension Society (Ramsay *et al.* 1999) now recommends that drug treatment should be considered for individuals with blood pressures of 140/90 mmHg and over. For young, middle-aged, diabetic hypertensive patients and patients with a history of MI, the levels should be <130/85 mmHg, and <140/90 mmHg for elderly patients. Lifestyle measures that have been shown to reduce blood pressure are reducing salt and alcohol intake where appropriate, weight loss, and to a lesser extent, stress control and exercise (Alderman 1994). Diets rich in fruit and vegetables and low in total and saturated fats may also lower blood pressure (Appel *et al.* 1997).

Conditional risk factors

Conditional risk factors are associated with an increased risk for CHD but there is uncertain evidence about causation. Such factors include elevated serum triglycerides, homocysteine and coagulation factors (e.g. fibrinogen and plasminogen activator inhibitor-1.) Homocysteine, a normal constituent of blood is produced by the catabolism of dietary proteins, and normal values are 7–14 mmol/l. Raised levels, however, are linked with CHD and stroke. This may be due to a deficiency of vitamin B12, B6 and folate causing hyperhomocysteinaemia, estimated to be present in 1–2% of the general population.

Because atherosclerosis is an inflammatory process (Ross 1999), several plasma markers of inflammation have also been evaluated as potential tools for prediction of the risk of CHD. These markers include C reactive protein, serum amyloid A and interleukin-6, and some of these inflammatory markers have shown significance in postmenopausal women (Ridker *et al.* 2000).

Predisposing risk factors

Predisposing factors may intensify the causal risk factors in some way and in CHD include:

- Obesity
- Physical inactivity
- Family history (e.g. of premature CHD)
- Gender
- Behavioural factors
- Socio-economic factors
- Ethnic factors
- Insulin resistance

Obesity

Despite the obsession with being slim, the prevalence of obesity within developed countries is increasing and a body mass index (BMI) greater than 25 is associated with increased blood pressure and an increase in cardiac and stroke mortality. About 46% of men and 32% of women are overweight (BMI of 25–30 kg/m^2) and a further 17% of men and 21% of women are obese (BMI of more than 30 kg/m^2) (Peterson & Rayner 2002). Body shape has taken on new significance, with an apple shape (android/central obesity) associated with increased risk of CHD compared with a more pear shaped (gynoid) body (Ashwell 1996). Calculating the waist-to-hip ratio to check for central obesity is a simple measure (waist divided by hip measurement) and should be less than 0.95 for men and 0.85 for women.

Physical inactivity

Society has changed in a number of ways not least in the amount of energy expended by individuals. Improved technology has revolutionised the way we work and play but increasingly this involves minimal physical exertion. It is estimated that only 37% of men and 25% of women in the UK are active enough to offer some protection against CHD. Of course people can delude themselves into believing they take adequate exercise, but for it to offer any advantage it needs to be of moderate intensity for at least 30 minutes on most days of the week (e.g. brisk walking, dancing or cycling).

Family history

Close relatives of patients with CHD have a 5–7-fold risk of eventually dying from heart disease and are more likely than relatives of healthy people to show signs such as arterial disease even before they develop symptoms. While this could indicate a genetic component of a disease, the importance of shared environmental factors such as diet cannot be discounted. Nevertheless, studies of identical and non-identical twins have provided useful data. Although both twins share the same environment, only identical twins share the same genes, and if a twin has CHD there is a 65% chance that an identical twin will have CHD (this is only 25% in a non-identical twin).

But how much of our behaviour is genetically determined? It has been suggested by Berg (1991) that genetic influences may determine an individual's ability to respond to behavioural modification of the physiological risk factors as well as determining the actual levels of the risk factors themselves.

Age and sex

It appears that fatty streaks in blood vessels appear very early on in life and in babies these are close to where arteries branch, probably due to turbulent blood flow. Although these disappear, they are evident again during adolescence. In men and women the death rate from CHD rises steeply with age, but up to the age of 45 years the number of male deaths is about five times that in women. In women the death rate from CHD lags behind that for men by about 10 years. Rates in women increase six-fold between the age groups of 35–44 and 45–54, i.e. before and after the menopause. This is similar to the increase in male death rates in the age groups 25–34 and 35–44. The number of deaths from CHD in women over 75 years is greater than in men of the same age. Some degree of protection against CHD in pre-menopausal women may be due to:

- Higher levels of HDL-cholesterol
- Lower iron stores
- Peripheral, rather than central fat distribution

An interesting longitudinal epidemiological study involved 84 129 nurses (women), who were free of diagnosed cardiovascular disease, cancer and diabetes when the study commenced in 1980. Over the next 14 years there were 1128 major coronary events (296 deaths from CHD and 832 non-fatal infarctions). In this study (Stampfer *et al.* 2000), overall risk seemed to be reduced in those women who:

- Did not smoke
- Were not overweight
- Maintained a healthy diet high in cereal fibre, omega-3 fatty acids, folate, high ratio of PUFA (polyunsaturated fatty acids) to saturated fat and low in trans fatty acids
- Exercised moderately or vigorously for half an hour each day
- Consumed alcohol moderately

The prognosis for women with heart disease is generally worse than for men. Until recently there was little research regarding CHD in women and this may have been due to the perception that women were protected against CHD and few were affected. With increased life expectancy the pattern has emerged showing this to be a serious problem for women also. It is likely that women with diabetes who also have other coronary risk factors may have increased risk for CHD as the mortality and morbidity rate for women is higher than in men with CHD and diabetes.

Psychosocial factors

Most would probably agree that psychosocial factors, not least stress, do in fact contribute in some way to the development of heart disease. Indeed there are those who believe that stress superimposed on other complex factors increases risk for most disease today. The concept of stress has been very difficult to operationalise in studies and this has hampered research in this area. Avoiding the term 'stress', Hemingway & Marmot (1999) reviewed the epidemiological literature which had explored the relevance of psychological factors in the development of heart disease and identified three possible pathways offering an explanation:

- Psychological factors may affect health-related behaviours such as smoking, diet, alcohol consumption or physical activity which may in turn influence the risk of coronary heart disease.
- Psychological factors may cause direct acute or chronic pathophysiological changes.
- Access to and content of social support may influence the link between social support and CHD.

Undoubtedly, there are many complex factors influencing behaviour, and health promotion involves far more than simply giving information. Social cognition theories explain how both social and environmental factors together with cognitions determine patterns of high risk behaviour. Plausible explanations have also been put forward regarding the link between ongoing chronic stress and the adverse physiological responses mainly mediated through the pituitary–adrenal axis and the possible development of cardiovascular events.

Personality typing

Personality typing has been a popular method of linking personality and behaviour, with individuals with Type A behaviour pattern (Friedman & Rosenman 1974) demonstrating:

- Aggression
- Competitiveness
- Chronic hurry
- Impatience
- Suppressed anger
- Hostility

However, findings in studies are very conflicting, not always showing an association between Type A behaviour patterns and heart disease. This is hardly surprising as dividing the population into two basic personality types is somewhat simplistic. What has emerged from the literature in this area is that hostility is one component of Type A personality which is likely to be significant, and has been shown to be a predictor for coronary events and mortality. Earlier work drew attention to the role of major negative life events, e.g. bereavement, migration and retirement, and their effect on cardiovascular risk. Perhaps of greater significance are the daily hassles (Kanner *et al.* 1981) experienced which result in ongoing frustration and stress. Not only are these concepts important when considering the development of CHD and other diseases, but their impact on individuals already coping with chronic illness also warrants further study. While short periods of acute stress need not be harmful, the impact of acute on chronic stress in vulnerable groups needs to be assessed.

Work-related stressors
Stressors encountered in the work situation have also been explored. Of significance here is the way we perceive our work with two factors being particularly important: perceived demand and control. Occupations where there are excessive demands being made on the individual who has very little control, usually jobs of low status, create environments where risk of disease development is increased. Conversely, jobs where there is high demand and high control are less stressful.

Social support
An important buffer it seems in all this, which helps people to cope with stressful circumstances is social support, or, more accurately, perceived social support. Social support is likely to be one of the most important factors determining whether or not someone copes effectively with chronic illness once discharged home. Social isolation is in itself a stressor which has been shown to contribute to risk in terms of disease susceptibility and mortality (Berkman & Syme 1979). In surveys, men (16%) are more likely to report a lack of social support than women (11%) (Joint Health Surveys Unit 1999). Family relationships and how people live are changing dramatically, with more and more people choosing to live alone and relatives living at a distance. While this poses few difficulties during early adulthood, with an ageing population we need to start thinking about how best to support the more vulnerable in society.

Social class differences

There are exceptions, but for most cardiac and respiratory diseases there is a social class gradient, with those in the lower socio-economic groups bearing most of the burden in terms of morbidity and mortality. The premature death rate from CHD is 58% higher for men who are manual workers than it is for non-manual workers. Although the rate is falling across all social groups, the rate of fall is greater in the non-manual groups (Petersen & Rayner 2002).

In the Whitehall Study of Civil Servants (Marmot *et al.* 1978), the lowest grade of employees had three times the mortality of men in the highest grades over the ten-year follow-up period. Although there were higher rates of smoking, obesity, raised blood pressure and less physical activity in the lower grades, these factors did not fully explain the differences in mortality between the groups.

Socio-economic disadvantage increases the risk of individuals on a number of levels including disease development, access to health care and recovery from surgery. Tackling inequalities in health is of importance in all countries and reduction in socio-economic variation in mortality from a number of diseases is likely to be best addressed by primary and secondary prevention.

Infant origins of disease

There is ongoing debate regarding the significance of adverse factors, including under-nutrition possibly affecting early development in utero. It is argued that factors acting in early life may have consequences for the later risk of certain diseases, including CHD (Barker 1992) and some respiratory diseases, e.g. COPD. Under-nutrition may permanently reduce the number of cells in particular organs and may also change:

- Distribution of cell types
- Patterns of hormonal secretion
- Metabolic activity
- Organ structure

Others argue that Barker's findings are due to bias because of selective migration and confounding variables linked with lifestyle during adulthood.

Ethnic group differences

Gujaratis, Punjabis, Bangladeshis and southern Indians in London have 40% higher CHD mortality rates than UK national averages (McKeigue *et al.* 1991). Similar findings have been found in a number of different countries around the world (e.g. Singapore, South Africa, Uganda and Fiji). The British Heart Foundation put the premature death rate in these groups (including Sri Lankans) at 46% higher for men and 51% higher for women.

Once more, differences in rates cannot be explained entirely by differences in diet, plasma cholesterol levels or smoking habits. In some Asian groups the smoking rate and cholesterol levels are lower than in the general population. There is evidence to suggest that increased prevalence of non-insulin diabetes mellitus, which in some Asian communities in London is four times the national average, may be responsible. Insulin resistance and central obesity are more common in Asian groups than in Europeans.

The risk of many diseases cannot be predicted from just one risk factor. CHD, for example, is a multifactorial disease, and while some combinations of risk factors seem to be especially important (e.g. smoking, cholesterol and high blood pressure), individual susceptibility is also an important factor.

This chapter has set the scene by outlining the prevalence of cardiorespiratory disease and identifying those groups where surgical intervention is an option. An exploration of key issues concerning the ongoing debate regarding risk factors further equips the surgical nurse working in a cardiothoracic setting with the requisite background knowledge to increase the effectiveness of her health promotion role. Other sections will explore other dimensions of health promotion in optimising the patient's health both before and following surgery.

References

Alderman, M.H. (1994) Non pharmacological treatment of hypertension. *Lancet* **344**: 307–11.

Appel, L.J., Moore, T.J., Obarzanek, E. *et al.* (1997) A clinical trial of the effects of dietary patterns on blood pressure. DASH Collaborative Research Group. *New England Journal of Medicine* **336**: 1117–24.

Ashwell, M. (1996) Leaping into shape. In: Sadler, M.J. (ed.) *Bodyweight and Health. Proceedings of the British Nutrition Foundation Conference.* British Nutrition Foundation, London.

Barker, D.J.P. (1992) *Fetal and infant origins of adult disease.* BMJ Publishing Group, London.

Berkman, L.F. & Syme, S.L. (1979) Social networks, host resistance and mortality: a nine year follow up study of Alameda County residents. *American Journal of Epidemiology* **109**: 186–204.

Berg, K. (1991) Interaction of nutrition and genetic factors in health and disease. Proceedings of 6th European Nutrition Conference. *European Journal of Clinical Nutrition* **45** (Suppl. 2): 8–13.

Bjortuft, O., Simonsen, S., Geiran, O.R. *et al.* (1996) Pulmonary haemodynamics after single lung transplantation for end stage pulmonary parenchymal disease. *European Respiratory Journal* **9**: 2007–11.

Bouros, D., Psathakis, K. & Siafakas, N.M. (1997) Quality of life in interstitial lung disease. *European Respiratory Review* **7**(42): 66–70.

British Lung Foundation (1996) *The Lung Report. Lung Disease: A Shadow over the Nation's Health.* British Lung Foundation, London.

British Thoracic Society (1997) BTS guidelines for the management of chronic obstructive pulmonary disease. *Thorax* **52** (Suppl. 5).

British Thoracic Society (2001) *The Burden of Lung Disease.* British Thoracic Society, London.

Cole, P. (1995) Bronchiectasis. In: Brewis, R.A.L., Corrin, B., Geddes, D.M. & Gibson, G.J. (eds) *Respiratory Medicine.* W.B. Saunders, London.

Criqui, M.H. & Ringel, B.L. (1994) Does diet or alcohol explain the French paradox? *Lancet* **344**: 1719–23.

Dawber, T.R. (1980) *The Framingham Study.* Harvard University Press, Cambridge MA.

Diaz, M.N., Frei, B., Vita, J.A. & Keaney, J.F. Jr (1997) Antioxidants and atherosclerotic heart disease. *New England Journal of Medicine* **337**(6): 408–16.

DoH (Department of Health) (1995) *Sensible Drinking. The Report of an Inter-departmental Working Group.* HMSO, London.

DoH (Department of Health) (1998) *Improving Outcomes in Lung Cancer. DoH manual 97CC122 and Research Evidence 97CC123.* HMSO, London.

Doll, R. & Peto, P. (1996) *Oxford Textbook of Medicine.* Oxford University Press, Oxford.

Doll, R., Peto, R., Wheatley, K. *et al.* (1994) Mortality in relation to smoking: 40 years observation on male British doctors. *British Medical Journal* **309**: 901–11.

du Bois, R.M. (1990) Cryptogenic fibrosing alveolitis. In: Brewis, R.A.L., Gibson, G.J. & Geddes, D.M. (eds) *Respiratory Medicine.* Baillière Tindall, London.

Edwards, J.G. & Waller, D.A. (2001) The evidence base for surgical intervention in lung cancer. In: Muers M.F., Macbeth, F., Wells, F.C. & Miles, A. (eds) *The Effective Management of Lung Cancer.* Aesculapius Medical Press, London.

Evans, M. & Rees, A. (2002) Does it matter which statin you choose? *Cardiabetes* **2**(2): 24–8.

Friedman, M. & Rosenman, R.H. (1974) *Type A Behaviour and Your Heart.* Alfred A. Knopf, New York.

Fulmer, J.D. (1982) An introduction to interstitial lung disease. *Clinical Chest Medicine* **3**: 257–64.

Grossman, R.F., Frost, A., Zamel N. *et al.* (1990) Results of single lung transplantation for bilateral pulmonary fibrosis. *New England Journal of Medicine* **322**: 727–33.

Grundy, S.M. (1999) Primary prevention of coronary heart disease: integrating risk assessment with intervention. *Circulation* **11**(9): 988–98.

Hanagiri, T., Muranaka, H., Hashimoto, M., Nagashima, A. & Yasumoto , K. (1999) Results of surgical treatment of lung cancer in octogenarians. *Lung Cancer* **23**: 129–33.

Hemingway, H. & Marmot, M. (1999) Evidenced based cardiology: psychosocial factors in the aetiology and prognosis of coronary heart disease: systematic review of prospective cohort studies. *British Medical Journal* **318**: 1460–67.

Hertog, M.G.L. (1993) Dietary antioxidant flavonoids and risk of coronary heart disease: the Zutphen Elderly Study. *Lancet* **342**: 1007–11.

Hosenpud, J.D., Bennett, LE., Keck, B.M. *et al.* (1998) Effect of diagnosis on survival benefit of lung transplantation for end-stage lung disease. *Lancet* **351**: 24–7.

Joint Health Surveys Unit (1999) *Health Survey for England 1998.* The Stationery Office, London.

Julian, D., Camm, J., Fox, K.M. & Poole-Wilson, P. (1996) *Diseases of the Heart*, 2nd edn. W.B. Saunders, London.

Kanner, A.D., Coyne, J.C., Schaeffer, C. & Lazarus, R.S. (1981) Comparison of two modes of stress measurement: daily hassles and uplifts versus major life events. *Journal of Behavioural Medicine* **4**: 1–39.

Law, M.R., Wald, N.J. & Thompson, S.G. (1994) By how much and how quickly does reduction in serum cholesterol concentration lower risk of ischaemic heart disease? *British Medical Journal* **308**: 367–72.

Lockhart, L., McMeeken, K. & Mark, J. (2000) Secondary prevention after myocardial infarction: reducing the risk of further cardiovascular events. *Coronary Health Care* **4**(2): 82–91.

Marmot, M.G. (1992) Primary prevention of stroke. *Lancet* **339**: 344–7.

Marmot, M.G., Rose, G., Shipley, M. & Hamilton, P.J. (1978) Employment grade and coronary heart disease in British civil servants. *Journal of Epidemiology and Community Health* **32**(4): 244–9.

McKeigue, P.M., Shah, B. & Marmot, M.G. (1991) Relation of central obesity and insulin resistance with high diabetes prevalence and cardiovascular risk in South Asians. *Lancet* **337**: 382–6.

Morgan, W.E. (1996) The surgical management of lung cancer. *British Journal of Hospital Medicine* **55**(10): 631–4.

Muers, M. (1995) Lung cancer. *Medicine* **23**(9): 361–9.

Mukamal, K., Maclure, M., Muller, J. *et al.* (2001) Prior alcohol consumption and mortality following acute myocardial infarction. *Journal of the American Medical Association* **285**(15): 1965–70.

Otto, C. (2002) Calcification of bicuspid aortic valves. *Heart* **88**(4): 321–2.

Pagni, S., McKelvey, A., Riordan, C., Federico, J.A. & Ponn, R.B. (1998) Pulmonary resection for malignancy in the elderly: is age still a risk factor? *European Journal of Cardio-Thoracic Surgery* **14**: 40–44.

Petersen, S. & Rayner, M. (2002) *Coronary Heart Disease Statistics*. British Heart Foundation, London.

Peto, R., Lopez, A.D., Boreham J., Thun, M., Heath, C. Jr, Doll, R. (1996) Mortality from smoking worldwide. *British Medical Bulletin* **52**(1): 12–21.

Ramsay, L., Williams, B., Johnston, G.D. *et al.* (1999) British Hypertension Society guidelines for hypertension management 1999: summary. *British Medical Journal* **319**: 630–35.

Ridker, P.M., Hennekens, C.H., Buring, J.E. & Rifai, N. (2000) C-reactive protein and other markers of inflammation in the prediction of cardiovascular disease in women. *New England Journal of Medicine* **342**(12): 836–43.

Ross, R. (1999) Atherosclerosis – an inflammatory disease. *New England Journal of Medicine* **340**: 115–26.

Shaper, A.G., Pocock, S.J. & Walker, M. (1981) British regional heart study: cardiovascular risk factors in middle aged men in 24 towns. *British Medical Journal* (Clinical Research Edition) **283**(6185): 179–86.

Stampfer, M.J., Hu, F.B., Manson, J.E. *et al.* (2000) Primary prevention of coronary heart disease in women through diet and lifestyle. *New England Journal of Medicine* **343**(1): 16–22.

Stavem, K., Bjortuft, O., Lund, M.B. *et al.* (2000) Health related quality of life in lung transplant candidates and recipients. *Respiration* **67**: 159–65.

Sulica, R., Teirstein, A. & Padilla, M.L. (2001) Lung transplantation in interstitial lung disease. *Current Opinion in Pulmonary Medicine* **7**(5): 314–21.

Tribble, D.L. (1999) Antioxidant consumption and risk of coronary heart disease: emphasis on vitamin C, vitamin E and beta carotene. *Circulation* **99**: 591–5.

Tunstall-Pedoe, H., Brown, C.A., Woodward, M. & Tavendale, R. (1995) Passive smoking by self report and serum cotinine and the prevalence of respiratory and coronary heart disease in the Scottish heart study. *Journal of Epidemiology and Community Health* **49**: 139–43.

Turner-Warwick, M., Burrows, B. & Johnson, A. (1980) Cryptogenic fibrosing alveolitis: clinical features and their influence on survival. *Thorax* **35**: 171–80.

Wilson, C.B., Jones P.W., O'Leary, C.J., Hansell, D.M., Cole, P.J. & Wilson, R. (1997) Effect of sputum bacteriology on the quality of life of patients with bronchiectasis. *European Respiratory Journal* **10**(8): 1754–60.

Wilson, P.W., D'Agostino, R.B., Levy, D. *et al.* (1998) Prediction of coronary heart disease using risk factor categories. *Circulation* **97**: 1837–47.

Further reading

British Heart Foundation Statistics Database 2002
www.heartstats.org
British Thoracic Society. *The Burden of Lung Disease: A Statistical Report.*
www.brit-thoracic.org.uk

Applied Respiratory and Cardiac Physiology

Following most cardiothoracic surgical procedures the patient's respiratory and haemodynamic status is invariably compromised to some degree. Obviously the more invasive the procedure the greater potential there is for instability. Effective tissue oxygenation is paramount and the skilled cardiothoracic nurse will need to be vigilant in monitoring a number of parameters in ensuring that cardiac and respiratory functioning is optimised. First, the lungs must be effectively ventilated in order that the pulmonary capillary blood may be oxygenated. Second, there must be an effective transport system in terms not only of adequate haemoglobin but also haemodynamic stability so that oxygenated blood is pumped effectively around the body.

Respiratory system

Hypoxaemia is common following surgery and develops because one or more of the processes leading to effective oxygenation of blood in the lungs is altered in some way. A good knowledge of these physiological processes will help the nurse to complete a comprehensive assessment and identify where in the chain problems are arising.

An overview of the respiratory system will be given with emphasis on the relationships between airways, lungs and chest wall. The effective dynamics of ventilation are dependent on a number of physical properties of the system and these will be considered. Processes occurring during ventilation will follow, including factors contributing to the control of breathing. Once the air in the lungs has been replenished then gases must diffuse across the alveolar–capillary surface and the last section will explore the transport of gases in the blood and the maintenance of acid-base status.

While the lungs have a number of functions, including acid–base balance, pulmonary defence and metabolism of many bioactive substances, the principal function is that of gaseous exchange. The respiratory system facilitates the intake of oxygen and the removal of carbon dioxide from the body. Oxygen must be available to the cells for the process of oxidative phosphorylation, an important process in aerobic metabolism. It is in the mitochondria that the high-energy phosphate bond in adenosine triphosphate (ATP) is produced from adenosine diphosphate (ADP). This ADP/ATP energy system is the most important system in the body. However, there are no stores of ATP in the body and it must be synthesised continuously as it is being used. The critical oxygen tension varies between organs, but a mitochondrial PO_2 of about 0.13 kPa (1 mmHg) is often considered the level below which there is a serious impairment of oxidative phosphorylation and a switch to anaerobic metabolism.

Aerobic metabolism is the most efficient source of biological energy. Although skeletal muscle can function for short periods under conditions of anaerobic metabolism this is not possible in organs such as the brain, liver and heart which require a continuous supply of oxygen. Carbon dioxide is a waste product of aerobic metabolism and the body must be able to remove this. The body at rest needs approximately 250 ml per minute of oxygen, and 200 ml of carbon dioxide per minute is removed. It is vital therefore that air be continuously exchanged between the lungs and atmosphere and the unique properties of the pulmonary system facilitate this.

Airways, lungs and chest wall

During inspiration air is filtered, warmed and moistened by the upper respiratory tract as it passes down the tracheobronchial tree. Figure 3.1 shows the various branches of the respiratory tree. Although patency of the larger airways is ensured by the presence of cartilage in their walls, in the smaller bronchioles (<1 mm diameter) cartilage is absent. It is mainly smooth muscle that is found here. The whole tracheobronchial tract is lined with ciliated columnar epithelium. Muco-ciliary function facilitates the upward removal of debris from the airways enabling the lower air spaces to remain relatively sterile.

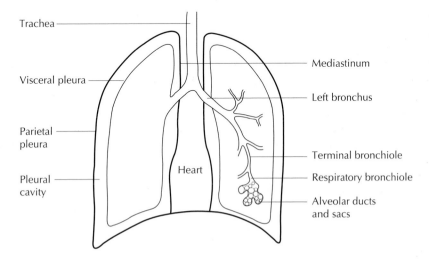

Fig. 3.1   Thoracic cavity with outline of respiratory tract.

Not all the air taken in with each breath (tidal volume) is available for gaseous exchange. Figure 3.2 shows the anatomical dead space, which includes the larger airways down to, and including, the terminal bronchioles. The last portion of the tidal volume (30%) remains in this anatomical dead space and is roughly equivalent to 2 ml/kg body weight, around 150 ml in an adult. In effect this is wasted ventilation which can be further increased when additional alveolar dead space occurs because of ventilated alveoli which have no perfusion. This alveolar dead space combined with the anatomical dead space is referred to as physiological dead space. An increase in physiological dead space does not usually cause concern until its volume is significant.

Generations 17 to 23 of the tracheobronchial tree are made up of respiratory bronchioles, alveolar ducts and alveolar sacs. Collectively, these structures comprise the acinus, referred to as the respiratory zone as the air in this section is available for gaseous exchange. Approximately 70% of the tidal volume (350 ml in adults) enters the respiratory zone and this volume over one minute is the alveolar volume.

The respiratory zone offers a huge surface area for gaseous exchange. Adult lungs contain around 300 million alveoli with a surface area between 60 and

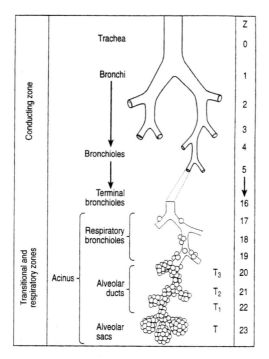

Fig. 3.2 Diagram of airway branching in the human lung. From Weibel (1963), with permission.

$100\,m^2$. Each alveolus is in contact with pulmonary capillaries having a diameter of only 12 microns, just enough to enable the passage of a red blood cell. Gas molecules must diffuse through a relatively complex layer of cells called the alveolar–capillary membrane (see Fig. 3.3). The wall of the alveoli is composed of the following:

- Type I pneumocytes – flat epithelial cells (97% of lining)
- Type II pneumocytes – large cuboidal cells rich in mitochondria which release surfactant
- Alveolar macrophages – derived from circulating monocytes and important in destroying foreign protein and pathogens

The alveolar–capillary membrane, despite its complexity is only 0.5 microns in thickness.

The lungs remain inflated and are prevented from collapsing because of the integrity of the pleural space. The mediastinum and chest wall are lined by parietal pleura and the lungs are covered by visceral pleura. The pleural cavity between these two pleural membranes is a potential space and the pressure is subatmospheric.

Throughout inspiration and expiration the pressure within the pleural cavity remains less than the pressure in the airways (transpulmonary pressure difference) and this is important in helping to keep the lungs inflated. Whenever pleural

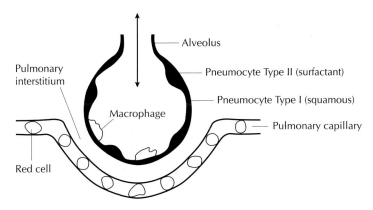

Fig. 3.3 Alveolar–capillary membrane.

pressure is the same or greater than atmospheric pressure (reduced transpulmonary pressure gradient) there is a danger of small airway collapse. Remember that there is no cartilage in the smaller bronchioles to maintain patency. Forced expiratory efforts such as coughing (producing more positive intrapleural pressure) following surgery may be counterproductive because when the transpulmonary pressure difference is reduced airway closure occurs.

Mechanism of breathing

Atmospheric air consists of a number of gases but mainly oxygen (20.98%), carbon dioxide (0.04%), and nitrogen (76%). Each gas in a mixture of gases exerts a pressure (partial pressure) independent of other gases present (Dalton's law) and the sum total of these partial pressures in air is called atmospheric or barometric pressure (P_B). The partial pressure of a gas is proportional to its fractional concentration and with an atmospheric pressure of 101 kPa at sea level the partial pressure is calculated as follows:

$$PO_2 = \frac{20.98}{100} \times 101 \text{ kPa} = 21.18 \text{ kPa}$$

However, when calculating the partial pressure of gases in the alveoli the fractional concentration of carbon dioxide and oxygen is different with oxygen constituting 14% of the gases. Water vapour also exerts a partial pressure (PH_2O), and at a body temperature of 37°C this is around 6 kPa. Therefore to calculate the partial pressure of oxygen, for example, in the alveoli, 6 kPa must be subtracted from 101 kPa (i.e. 95 kPa). Thus:

$$\text{Alveolar } PO_2 \ (PAO_2) = \frac{14}{100} \times 95 \text{ kPa} = 13.3 \text{ kPa}$$

Air must be continuously replenished in the lungs and this is achieved by volume/pressure changes in the thoracic cavity during inspiration and expiration. The ribs, intercostal muscles, diaphragm and chest wall are all important in bringing about these changes.

An understanding of normal adult lung volumes is necessary in order to appreciate the changes which occur when pulmonary status is compromised. Figure 3.4 demonstrates a typical spirometry trace and identifies the various lung volumes. Tidal volume (TV) is the amount of air breathed in and out with each breath and is approximately 500 ml in an adult. Multiplying this volume by the number of breaths per minute (RR) yields the minute or pulmonary volume, approximately 6 litres at rest. Not all this volume is available for gaseous exchange, and subtracting the dead space (DS) volume from tidal volume gives the alveolar volume (AV), approximately 4 litres at rest:

$$AV = RR \times (TV - DS)$$

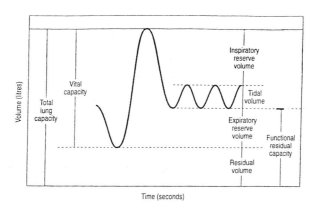

Fig. 3.4   Lung volumes.

Maintaining effective alveolar ventilation ensures that PaO_2 and $PaCO_2$ remain within acceptable parameters. For example, if alveolar ventilation is halved then $PaCO_2$ is doubled. A rising $PaCO_2$ is called hypercapnia and a fall in PaO_2 hypoxaemia.

Inspiration is initiated as a result of rising levels of carbon dioxide in arterial blood ($PaCO_2$) and therefore cerebrospinal fluid (CSF). An increase in hydrogen ions stimulates the central chemoreceptors in the medulla oblongata resulting in neuronal discharge to muscles involved in breathing. As a result of muscle contraction there is an increase in both the lateral and anteroposterior diameters of the thorax. According to Boyle's law, at a constant temperature, pressure is inversely proportional to volume, so as the thoracic cavity increases, alveolar pressure (and pleural pressure) decreases (relative to atmospheric pressure) and air enters the lungs. Expiration involves passive recoil of the alveoli and intrapleural pressure becomes less negative once more.

The work of breathing

Breathing usually involves very little effort, but energy must nevertheless be expended to overcome opposing forces during inspiration. The effort required to overcome these opposing forces is called the work of breathing, where muscular contraction is required to distend the elastic tissues of the chest wall and lungs (elastic work or compliance work) and to move air through the respiratory passages (resistance work). The work of breathing may increase considerably following surgery owing to a number of factors. The increased muscle contraction will increase oxygen consumption, further compromising the cardiopulmonary system and oxygen delivery. Knowledge of the factors contributing to the work of breathing is therefore important.

Compliance work

Most of the work of breathing is necessary to overcome the elastic recoil of the lungs and chest wall (65% of the work). Both the chest wall and lung tissue contribute to total compliance. Pulmonary tissue tends to recoil inwards and the chest wall recoils outwards. There must be a pressure change to move air into the lungs. Distensibility or compliance refers to the ability of the lungs to increase volume and the chest wall to move to accommodate this increase. It is a measure of the lung's opposition to inflation and is the inverse of elastance (elastic recoil), which is the ease with which something can be stretched. The more elastic the lung then the less compliant (stiffer) it is.

Most surgical nurses will not have access to data on compliance, but factors which may be decreasing compliance and increasing the work of breathing necessitating greater inspiratory effort need to be considered. Chest deformity and obesity may reduce compliance as will pathology such as pulmonary fibrosis, pulmonary oedema and pneumothorax. In these cases, lung compliance is low and greater transpulmonary pressures need to be generated during inspiration to move air into the lungs. The presence of incisional pain, drains, restrictive dressings and bedclothes may all decrease compliance and the patient may breathe at low lung volumes. Although the lungs are usually more compliant at lower volumes and less compliant at higher volumes it is difficult to inflate alveoli that are closed and much greater inspiratory pressures are required to open them.

Interestingly, in emphysema compliance is increased. However, there is a reduction in elastance so that removing air from the lungs during expiration is more difficult (air trapping results).

Surface tension in the alveoli

Another factor which influences the volume–pressure behaviour of the lung is the surface tension created at the air–liquid interface of the alveoli. Such surface tension always occurs whenever a gas and liquid come into contact with each other generating a cohesive force inwards. This surface tension in the alveoli contributes to collapse and once this occurs very high distending pressures are needed to reopen them (Savov 1995). Smaller alveoli are potentially very unstable, generate greater pressures and empty into larger alveoli resulting in collapse. This tendency is prevented by the presence of pulmonary surfactant which decreases surface tension dramatically as alveolar volume decreases.

Pulmonary surfactant is manufactured by pneumocyte type II cells and is a complex substance – 90% phospholipid and 10% protein. Palmitoyl phosphatidylcholine (DPPC) comprises about 50% of the phospholipid content. In summary, surfactant stabilises alveoli, increases compliance and reduces the work of breathing. It also reduces slightly the hydrostatic pressure in the interstitial fluid surrounding the alveoli therefore discouraging the movement of water from the capillaries and helps to keep the alveoli 'dry'. Problems with surfactant production following cardiothoracic surgery may contribute to alveolar collapse and micro-atelectasis in the early post-operative period.

Resistance work

Airway resistance
Another factor that influences the work of breathing is the degree of resistance to airflow and this is greater in the larger central airways. Airway resistance may be expressed as follows:

$$\text{Airway resistance} = \frac{\text{Driving pressure}}{\text{Flow rate}}$$

The driving pressure is the pressure gradient between the mouth and alveoli. At the end of expiration there is no airflow and atmospheric and alveolar pressures are the same. It is during inspiration that a pressure gradient exists, with alveolar pressure being less than atmospheric pressure creating the driving pressure for airflow into the lungs. During expiration the gradient is reversed so that alveolar exceeds mouth (atmospheric pressure) pressure and air flows out of the lung.

It is the diameter of a tube which most influences the flow of gas molecules. The greater the diameter the less chance there is of molecules colliding with the tube's wall. Increasing the length of a tube by 50% doubles airway resistance whereas if the radius is halved then resistance increases 16 times.

Many factors in health and disease can increase and decrease airway resistance. Although the small bronchioles have the smallest radius these airways are arranged in parallel so the total resistance offered by the millions of airways is quite low during normal quiet breathing. The medium-sized bronchi (2–4 mm diameter) are the site where there is important physiological control of airway resistance. Although these bronchi still have some supporting cartilage there is a great deal of smooth muscle that can contract to reduce the radius of the airways. Sputum plugs and the presence of endotracheal tubes and suction catheters can increase resistance further.

Resistance to airflow and airway closure
During both inspiratory and expiratory phases of breathing a transpulmonary (transmural) pressure difference exists whereby alveolar pressure remains greater than the subatmospheric pressure in the pleural cavity. This gradient assists in keeping the alveoli open by applying traction. However, high levels of airflow during forced expiration may cause reversal of the positive transpulmonary pressure difference (i.e. a negative transmural pressure) whereby the pressure in the lumen of the air passages becomes less than pleural cavity pressure resulting in dynamic airway compression. Forced expiratory efforts therefore may be

counterproductive particularly in patients with respiratory problems. Interestingly, patients with obstructive airways disease may acquire the habit of pursed lip breathing which will preserve the transmural pressure gradient in the airways, reduce airway resistance and therefore prevent air trapping.

Volume-related airway collapse

As the lung volume is reduced towards residual volume, there is a point at which lower dependent airways begin to close; this is known as the closing volume (CV). Usually in young adults, closing volume is well below functional residual capacity (FRC) so that closure only occurs at very low volumes. With increasing age the closing volume is nearer the FRC and airway closure can occur at much higher volumes particularly in the presence of lung disease. The elderly requiring surgery, therefore, may be particularly vulnerable. Furthermore, FRC is affected by positioning, decreasing from the upright to the supine position. Closure of airways will result in the shunting of blood through these areas, and is an important cause of hypoxaemia following cardiac and thoracic surgery as a result of atelectasis (Brismar *et al*. 1985).

If airway closure persists post-operatively it may be beneficial to increase lung volume. This is most conveniently achieved by the application of CPAP (continuous positive airway pressure) to the spontaneously breathing patient and PEEP (positive end expiratory pressure) in the ventilated patient which has the effect of increasing FRC so that airway closure is less likely.

Early ambulation and avoidance of the supine position will also help maintain FRC and post-operative oxygenation (Mynster *et al*.1996).

Airway epithelium

The tracheobronchial tree is lined with mucus-secreting epithelium and the function of this airway epithelium is more complex than once thought. Many of the epithelial cells are ciliated, with each cell housing over 200 cilia which beat around 1300 times per minute. A complex layer of mucus sits on top of the cilia and mucociliary activity is an important defence which protects the lower airway. This mechanism may be impaired in surgical patients due to smoking and the result of anaesthesia. Pre-existing pulmonary pathology will also increase the risk of pooling and stagnation of secretions.

The presence of immunoglobulins (Ig) or antibodies released by B lymphocytes, which is part of the humoral immune response, offers an additional defence mechanism in the airways. Secretory IgA is important in protecting mucous membranes, and a deficiency of immunoglobulins as a result of either primary or secondary causes can result in recurrent respiratory infections. IgE is an antibody which contributes to the development of allergic responses in atopic individuals (see below).

Other cells in the mucosal layers

In addition to epithelial cells, other cells with varying degrees of activity are found in the mucosal and submucosal layers. Eosinophils and neutrophils are polymorphonuclear leucocytes which migrate from the circulatory system to the airways. Eosinophils are found in great numbers in allergic asthma, whereas neutrophils are increased in chronic obstructive pulmonary disease and bacterial infections. Mast cells involved in allergic responses are found near the epithelial surface and contain histamine which, when released in the airways, causes bronchoconstriction and vasodilatation. In addition, mast cells along with other pro-inflammatory cells can synthesise a number of inflammatory mediators such as prostaglandins and thromboxane, which are the result of the breakdown of arachidonic acid in the cell membrane. Many of these mediators also result in bronchoconstriction and vasodilation.

Cytokines are cell messengers enabling cells to communicate with each other and many are chemotactic (chemokines) attracting other cells to areas of inflammation. Although cytokines have a key role to play in the inflammatory response, in some pathological conditions, e.g. acute respiratory distress syndrome (ARDS), they have been implicated as pro-inflammatory mediators. Primary pro-inflammatory cytokines are tumour necrosis factor (TNF α) and the interleukins (ILs) with IL-1 stimulating the release of IL-6 and IL-8. These cytokines together with other mediators such as thromboxane, leukotrienes and prostaglandins, give rise to a complex network which may initiate and amplify the inflammatory response in acute lung injury. It has been suggested that overdistension coupled with repeated collapse of alveoli in the ventilated patient may initiate a cascade of pro-inflammatory cytokines (Slutsky & Tremblay 1998).

Neurohormonal mechanisms

Neurohormonal mechanisms also have an important role in airway regulation. Autonomic neural control of the airways is by way of parasympathetic and sympathetic nerve fibres. Parasympathetic nerves, branches of the vagus nerve, release the neurotransmitter acetylcholine which results in smooth muscle contraction and therefore smaller lumen size. These cholinergic nerves exert their effects on muscarinic receptors causing contraction of smooth muscle (bronchoconstriction) and secretion of mucus from the submucosal glands and goblet cells. Drugs such as atropine sulphate, scopolamine and ipratropium bromide may be given to block these receptors and are therefore called anticholinergic or antimuscarinic agents.

Sympathetic nerves supply a number of different target organs where the neurotransmitter released is norepinephrine. However, sympathetic effects are also mediated by epinephrine and norepinephrine (hormones) released from the adrenal medulla. The sympathetic effect which these molecules exert will depend on the specific adrenergic receptor site on the cell membrane. Smooth muscle cells in the airways have β_2 receptors and have the potential to be stimulated by norepinephrine and epinephrine resulting in muscle relaxation and bronchodilation (Barnes 1986). Pharmacological agents acting on the β_2 receptors also relax the smooth muscle resulting in bronchodilation. These drugs are called β_2 agonists and examples are salbutamol and terbutaline.

A third branch of nerves supplying the airways has been identified called non-adrenergic non-cholinergic (NANC) nerves which can either be inhibitory (dilate) or excitatory (constrict). Inhibitory NANC nerves run in the vagus nerve and the neurotransmitters have been identified as vasoactive intestinal polypeptide (VIP) (Barnes *et al.* 1991) and nitric oxide (NO) (Belvisi *et al.* 1992) although NO appears to be the major neurotransmitter for bronchodilation.

Nitric oxide was originally identified as the endothelial relaxing factor (EDRF) but is in fact released by many different cells in the body, including airway epithelium. It is oxidised very quickly, has a half-life of less than 5 seconds (Al-Ali & Howarth 1998) and has a variety of physiological functions in almost all body systems. Although beneficial, it is in fact a free radical and can be toxic resulting in cell damage (Sadeghi Hashjin *et al.* 1996).

Additional nerve fibres in the airways include a number of sensory nerves and receptors in the airways, e.g. non-myelinated C-fibres. Receptors include stretch receptors, irritant receptors and C-fibre receptors. Sensory C-fibre receptors are sensitive to inflammatory mediators such as bradykinin, histamine and prostaglandins (Spina 1996). A number of neuropeptides including substance P are released by sensory nerves and these have been shown to increase airway responsiveness in asthma (Joos *et al.* 1995).

Pulmonary blood flow

The bronchial arteries are part of the systemic circulation and branch off the descending aorta. They supply oxygen and nutrients to all respiratory structures down to and including the terminal bronchioles. The respiratory bronchioles receive oxygen and nutrients from the pulmonary capillaries. A proportion of the bronchial venous blood draining the lungs empties into the azygos veins and then the pulmonary veins. This venous blood added to the oxygenated blood in the pulmonary veins represents a small anatomical shunt which is around 1–2% of the cardiac output (Q_t).

Pulmonary circulation

Ventilation of the lungs alone does not facilitate the diffusion of gas molecules. The pulmonary capillaries supply the alveoli and are an important part of the alveolar capillary membrane across which gaseous exchange takes place. Deoxygenated blood from the right side of the heart enters the pulmonary artery (referred to as mixed venous blood) and branches to form pulmonary capillary networks. Here the blood is oxygenated and returned via the pulmonary veins to the left atrium.

The flow of blood through the pulmonary circulation is approximately equal to the flow through the whole of the systemic circulation varying from around 6 l/min under resting conditions to as much as 25 l/min in severe exercise. Increases in flow are possible through the recruitment of additional blood vessels. The pulmonary circulation therefore is a low-pressure, low-resistance, high-volume system with pulmonary arterial pressure about one sixth of systemic arterial pressure (20 mmHg systolic and 8 mmHg diastolic).

Control of pulmonary vasomotor tone

There are many mediators which have a vasoactive role and some of these are outlined in the section on cardiovascular regulation later in this chapter. In response to hypoxia, blood vessels in the body mostly dilate. Pulmonary vessels, however, constrict in response to low levels of oxygen. Constriction occurs, for example, when the partial pressure of oxygen in the alveolus (PAO_2) is low. This mechanism is called hypoxic pulmonary vasoconstriction (HPV) and the major effects are the redistribution of blood away from poorly ventilated areas to alveoli that are better ventilated and a rise in pulmonary artery pressure. This appears to be a local reflex response occurring only in areas of alveolar hypoxia and occurs in surgically removed, mechanically perfused lungs demonstrating that there is no nervous or humoral dependency (Beachey 1998).

It should be noted that a number of drugs may also have an effect on vasomotor tone in the pulmonary circulation. A fall in PaO_2, for example, may be seen with the β agonists dopamine and dobutamine which increase blood flow to poorly ventilated areas (Rennotte *et al.* 1989). Dobutamine inhibits the HPV response whereas dopamine vasoconstricts blood vessels in the oxygenated lung thus decreasing the flow diversion from the hypoxic area by increasing the pulmonary artery pressure (Nomoto & Kawamura 1989). Vasodilators such as nitroglycerine and sodium nitroprusside may also result in arterial hypoxaemia during administration most likely due to an increase in NO release resulting in an increased shunt because of inhibition of the HPV response (D'Oliveira *et al.* 1981).

Ventilation–perfusion relationships

Ideally, lung ventilation (V) would match perfusion (Q), but this is not the case. In health there are regional variations in the ventilation–perfusion relationship and varying degrees of mismatching are common in pulmonary disorders. Indeed, one of the most common causes of hypoxaemia is ventilation–perfusion mismatch. When discussing the $\dot{V}/\dot{Q}$ relationship, $\dot{V}$ refers to the volume of gas per unit of time (per minute) which is alveolar ventilation, and $\dot{Q}$ is blood flow (perfusion) per unit of time (per minute) which is cardiac output. At rest, alveolar ventilation is around 4.21 per minute and perfusion is 5 l per minute.

In the upright position, gravitational forces and the characteristics of the pulmonary circulation result in regional variations not only of perfusion but also of ventilation. In the apices ventilation is greater than perfusion at rest and the converse is true in the bases. Despite these differences, in health there is greater overall ventilation and perfusion in the bases with corresponding greater gaseous exchange.

Where there is some pulmonary abnormality due to pathology or as a result of surgery, $\dot{V}/\dot{Q}$ relationships may change and this is illustrated in Fig. 3.5. A common cause of hypoxaemia following cardiothoracic surgery is where some alveoli receive too little ventilation compared with blood flow (low $\dot{V}/\dot{Q}$). A shunt-like effect occurs where pulmonary capillary blood in the affected area is not oxygenated. This is referred to as venous admixture and represents a proportion of the cardiac output which has bypassed the lungs. This may be partial

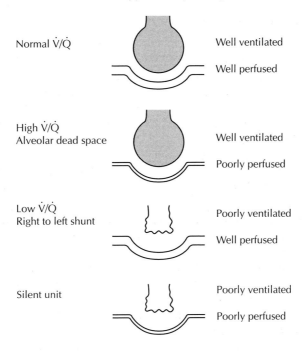

Normal $\dot{V}/\dot{Q}$	Well ventilated
	Well perfused
High $\dot{V}/\dot{Q}$ Alveolar dead space	Well ventilated
	Poorly perfused
Low $\dot{V}/\dot{Q}$ Right to left shunt	Poorly ventilated
	Well perfused
Silent unit	Poorly ventilated
	Poorly perfused

Fig. 3.5 Ventilation and perfusion relationships.

where there is some ventilation as in pulmonary oedema and bronchial asthma. When ventilation to a lung unit stops completely then there is an absolute right to left shunt and this can occur post-operatively when atelectasis or pneumonia develops. Although arterial PO_2 can be restored to normal with shunts up to about 30% by an appropriate increase in the inspired oxygen concentration, absolute shunts are often refractory to oxygen therapy.

Transport of gases

Once the alveolar air has been replenished, conditions must exist in the alveoli so that oxygen molecules are able to diffuse across the alveolar capillary membrane into pulmonary capillary blood and carbon dioxide molecules diffuse in the opposite direction. It is Fick's law which explains the diffusion of gases across the alveolar capillary membrane where rate of diffusion is directly proportional to surface area, diffusion coefficient (solubility and molecular weight), pressure gradient and inversely proportional to membrane thickness.

Although oxygen is not as soluble as carbon dioxide its molecular weight is lower and, according to Graham's law, rate of diffusion of a gas is inversely proportional to its molecular weight. Diffusion is also influenced by Henry's law which states that the amount of gas dissolved in a liquid is directly proportional to its partial pressure in the gas phase. This can be seen when the fractional inspired oxygen is increased achieving a much greater PAO_2 and therefore PaO_2.

A pressure gradient exists for the diffusion of oxygen because the $P\bar{v}O_2$ (mixed venous blood) is 5.3 kPa and the PAO_2 is 13 kPa. Oxygen molecules therefore diffuse across the alveolar–capillary membrane and into the pulmonary capillary blood. A pressure gradient also facilitates the diffusion of carbon dioxide from the pulmonary capillary blood into the alveoli. It takes each red blood cell approximately 0.75 seconds to traverse the pulmonary capillary surrounding the alveolus while equilibrium between alveolar and capillary PO_2 is achieved in just 0.25 seconds at rest.

With a normal PaO_2, only 3% of oxygen is carried dissolved in the plasma (around 0.3 ml/100ml), whereas 97% is chemically bonded to haemoglobin (Hb).

Oxyhaemoglobin

Haemoglobin is a combination of iron (haem) and protein (globin) but there are many different kinds of haemoglobin. Haemoglobin A is normal adult haemoglobin and for each molecule there are four sites which can carry four molecules of oxygen (oxyhaemoglobin). It is the proportion of sites carrying oxygen (i.e. saturation) which is measured by oximetry and usually this is around 97% in arterial blood and 75% in mixed venous blood. Desaturated blood is where the haemoglobin sites carry no oxygen.

$$Hb_4 + 4O_2 \Leftrightarrow Hb_4O_8$$

Oxygen capacity

When the haemoglobin is fully saturated (100%), each gram of haemoglobin can hold 1.39 ml of oxygen and this is called the oxygen capacity. The value for haemoglobin is normally around 15 g of haemoglobin in each 100 ml (d/l) of blood. The maximum amount of oxygen that can be combined with haemoglobin in every 100 ml of blood is therefore:

$$15 \times 1.39 = 20 \text{ ml } O_2/100 \text{ ml blood}$$

In the lungs, with a partial pressure of oxygen (PAO_2) of 13 kPa this will result in an arterial oxygen partial pressure (PaO_2) of 13 kPa. With a normal $PaCO_2$, pH and temperature, there should be around 19.5 ml of oxygen carried by haemoglobin in each 100 ml of blood for a saturation of 97.5%. Emptying of a small volume of bronchial venous blood into the pulmonary veins represents an anatomical shunt and this slightly desaturates the blood returning to the left ventricle.

To summarise, oxygen capacity is dependent upon PO_2 and level of haemoglobin.

Oxygen content

Oxygen content refers to the actual amount of oxygen attached to haemoglobin and dissolved in plasma and will be determined by the partial pressure of oxygen in the alveoli and arterial blood and the ability of haemoglobin molecules to combine with oxygen. In the following formula the small amount of dissolved oxygen in plasma is omitted.

$$\text{Arterial oxygen content (CaO}_2) = \frac{\text{Sat of Hb}}{100} \times O_2 \text{ capacity of Hb}$$

For example,

$$\frac{97}{100} \times (13 \times 1.39) = 17.5 \text{ ml/100 ml}$$

Knowing the arterial–mixed venous oxygen content difference $[C(a - \bar{v})O_2]$ enables the calculation of O_2 consumption (VO_2). For example,

$$\begin{aligned} VO_2 = Q_T \times C \ (19.5 - 14.5)O_2 &= 5 \text{ l/min} \times 5 \text{ ml/100 ml} \\ &= 5 \text{ l/min} \times 0.05 \\ &= 0.25 \text{ l/min} \\ &= 250 \text{ ml/min} \end{aligned}$$

Given the above it becomes clear that out of the usual 19.5 ml of oxygen available in every 100 ml of blood only approximately 5 ml (0.25) is released to the tissues, and this is referred to as the oxygen extraction ratio (O_2ER). At rest there is therefore an excess of supply over demand. With a resting cardiac output of 5000 ml, although around 1000 ml of oxygen is delivered per minute only 250 ml is used.

The maintenance of adequate oxygen delivery (DO_2) is an important goal following cardiothoracic surgery. Oxygen consumption (VO_2) and O_2ER will be increased when cardiac output falls or when there is an increase in oxygen demand, e.g. exercise, pyrexia and shivering post-operatively. Where demand is increased it is important to ensure that the supply (DO_2) can be maintained. Figure 3.6 illustrates oxygen delivery and consumption. Failure to ensure that delivery can meet increased demand can result in cellular hypoxia which may prove irreversible.

It is only in the critical care setting that VO_2 and DO_2 are calculated and this is usually based on cardiac index (CI) taking into account individual surface area which gives a more accurate estimate than cardiac output.

Oxyhaemoglobin dissociation curve

The chemical reaction between oxygen and haemoglobin is defined by the oxyhaemoglobin dissociation curve which relates the saturation of haemoglobin to the PaO_2. The shape of the curve has important physiological implications in that as the PaO_2 increases so does the affinity of haemoglobin for oxygen. The top, flat portion of the curve represents conditions in the lung where a PaO_2 of 13 kPa corresponds to an Hb saturation of 97.5% (Fig. 3.7).

The shape of the curve is sigmoid which is physiologically advantageous because the flat upper portion allows oxygen saturation to remain high and almost constant despite fluctuations in arterial PaO_2. Even with a PaO_2 of 8 kPa

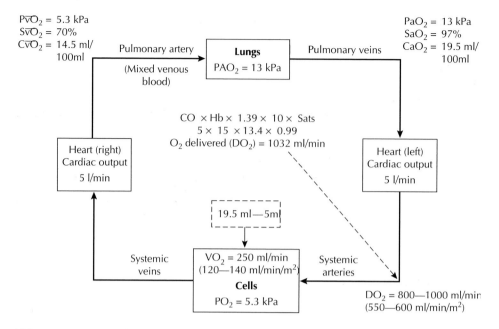

$P\bar{v}O_2$ = 5.3 kPa
$S\bar{v}O_2$ = 70%
$C\bar{v}O_2$ = 14.5 ml/
100ml

Pulmonary artery

(Mixed venous blood)

Lungs
PAO_2 = 13 kPa

Pulmonary veins

PaO_2 = 13 kPa
SaO_2 = 97%
CaO_2 = 19.5 ml/
100ml

CO × Hb × 1.39 × 10 × Sats
5 × 15 × 13.4 × 0.99
O_2 delivered (DO_2) = 1032 ml/min

Heart (right)
Cardiac output
5 l/min

Heart (left)
Cardiac output
5 l/min

19.5 ml—5ml

Systemic veins

VO_2 = 250 ml/min
(120—140 ml/min/m²)

Cells

PO_2 = 5.3 kPa

Systemic arteries

DO_2 = 800—1000 ml/min
(550—600 ml/min/m²)

Fig. 3.6 Oxygen delivery (DO_2) and consumption (VO_2) at rest. (DO_2 and VO_2 values are also given based on cardiac index.)

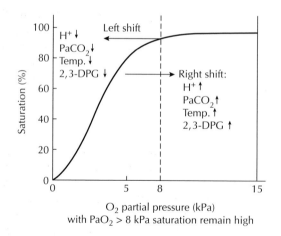

Fig. 3.7 Oxyhaemoglobin dissociation curve.

saturation remains 90% although below this desaturation occurs quickly. The steep segment of the curve enables large quantities of oxygen to be released in the peripheral capillaries.

There are a number of factors which may shift the position of the curve, altering the affinity of the haemoglobin. This response affects the pick-up and delivery of oxygen. The position of the normal curve shows the affinity of haemoglobin for oxygen when the following are normal:

- Temperature
- pH (or hydrogen ion concentration)
- Carbon dioxide
- Increased 2,3-diphosphoglycerate (2,3-DPG) in red blood cells (during hypoxia)

Figure 3.7 identifies factors which can shift the curve to either the left (greater affinity between haemoglobin and oxygen with less oxygen released) or to the right (less affinity between haemoglobin and oxygen with more oxygen released).

> To assess whether oxygen is being delivered satisfactorily, the following should be considered:
>
> - PAO_2 and PaO_2
> - Functional haemoglobin
> - Cardiac output
> - Unloading of oxygen

Cyanosis

The colour of blood depends on the amount of haemoglobin without oxygen (reduced haemoglobin). The skin will appear bluish when the capillary blood in it contains about 5 g/100 ml of haemoglobin in this form. However, central cyanosis may be detectable with lower levels of reduced haemoglobin. Cyanosis may be an unreliable indicator of tissue hypoxia. Anaemic patients can be severely hypoxic without cyanosis and polycythaemic patients with excess haemoglobin may be cyanosed with little hypoxia.

Carbon dioxide transport

Carbon dioxide is produced as a result of cell metabolism and this must be removed and transported to the lungs to be exhaled. This is achieved because carbon dioxide in solution moves down a pressure gradient from cell to extracellular fluid, plasma, red cell and finally alveoli. Like oxygen, most of the carbon dioxide is dissolved in plasma (70%) and chemically combined in the red cell (30%). The combined form of carbon dioxide may be carried as carbonic acid (10%), with protein as carbamino haemoglobin and plasma proteins (20%) and also as bicarbonate (70%).

Carbon dioxide partial pressure and content

It is interesting to compare the oxygen content and pressure with that of carbon dioxide in arterial and venous blood (see Table 3.1).

In the red cell, carbon dioxide (CO_2) combines with water (H_2O) to form carbonic acid (H_2CO_3) and this hydration of carbon dioxide is facilitated by an

Table 3.1 Differences in arterial and venous content and partial pressure of O_2 and CO_2

	Arterial	Venous
Oxygen	Content = 19.5 ml/100 ml PaO_2 = 13.0 kPa	Content = 14.5 ml/100 ml PvO_2 = 5.3 kPa
Carbon dioxide	Content = 48 ml/100 ml $PaCO_2$ = 4.6–6.0 kPa	Content = 52 ml/100 ml $PvCO_2$ = 5.5–6.8 kPa

enzyme called carbonic anhydrase which speeds the process up considerably. The carbonic acid which is formed dissociates into hydrogen ions (H^+) and bicarbonate ions (HCO_3^-) as follows:

$$CO_2 + H_2O \Leftrightarrow H_2CO_3 \Leftrightarrow HCO_3^- + H^+$$

The hydrogen ions attach themselves to the haemoglobin to form reduced haemoglobin which will become part of the carbamino compound. Although plasma proteins are able to take up hydrogen, haemoglobin has three times greater the affinity for carbon dioxide.

The bicarbonate (HCO_3^-) formed in the cell diffuses out through the cell membrane and moves into the plasma (see Fig. 3.8). Here it combines with sodium (Na^+) to form sodium bicarbonate ($NaHCO_3$). Because there is a loss of negative ions from the cell, to offset this there is a movement of chloride ions (Cl^-) into the cell to re-establish electrical neutrality. This is called the chloride shift.

When the blood reaches the lungs and flows through the pulmonary capillaries the reverse process takes place along with a reversal in the chloride shift:

$$H^+ + HCO_3^- \Leftrightarrow H_2CO_3 \Leftrightarrow H_2O + CO_2 \ (\uparrow exhaled)$$

Just as not all oxygen delivered to the tissues is unloaded, not all the carbon dioxide that diffuses from tissues and cells into the blood is eliminated in the lungs. Only a little carbon dioxide is eliminated with each breath – just enough to lower the $PaCO_2$ from 5.5.to 4.6 kPa.

When deoxygenation of the blood occurs at tissue level the loading of carbon dioxide is encouraged and this is called the Haldane effect. The lower the oxygen saturation then the more carbon dioxide that can be picked up at any given PCO_2. Conversely, when carbon dioxide combines with haemoglobin this encourages the release of oxygen, which is called the Bohr effect.

Acid–base balance

Many cellular processes require that the pH of body fluids is kept within a range which promotes normal tissue and organ performance. The pH scale is a measure of the degree of acidity/alkalinity of a solution, and arterial blood gas analysis in the early post-operative period following cardiothoracic surgery enables the

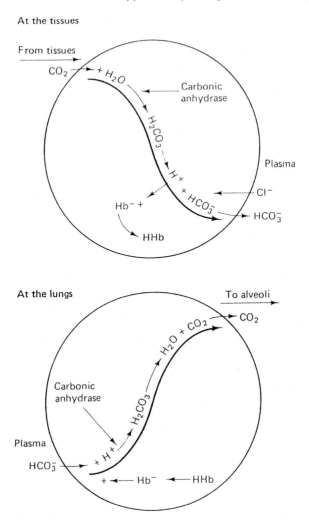

Fig. 3.8 Transport of carbon dioxide. From Widdicombe & Davies (1983), with permission.

monitoring of acid–base status (see Table 3.2 for normal values). In arterial blood the normal range for pH is 7.35–7.45, with the lower figure denoting more hydrogen ions (greater acidity) and the higher figure fewer hydrogen ions (greater alkalinity). Many units now measure hydrogen ion concentration, which offers a more linear scale, and the normal range is 35–45 nmol/l. This time the lower number denotes fewer hydrogen ions (more alkaline) and the higher figure more hydrogen ions (more acid).

The acid–base status of the body depends mainly on the ratio of dissolved carbon dioxide (quantified as $PaCO_2$) and HCO_3^- (bicarbonate). The ratio of HCO_3^- to $PaCO_2$ should be 20:1. It is when this ratio changes that a state of acidosis or alkalosis can occur. For example, a respiratory acidosis may arise because of an increase in $PaCO_2$ where the lungs are unable to remove carbon

Table 3.2 Acid-base balance – normal values

	Arterial blood	Venous blood
pH	7.35–7.45	7.31–7.41
Hydrogen ions	35–45 nmol/l	
PO_2	12–14 kPa	4.6–5.8 kPa
PCO_2	4.5–6.0 kPa	5.5–6.8 kPa
HCO_3	22–26 mmol/l	22–26 mmol/l
O_2	95%	70–75%
Base excess/deficit	-2 to $+2$	-2 to $+2$

dioxide effectively as in ventilatory failure. As carbon dioxide is released by the cells it is hydrated to carbonic acid (H_2CO_3). This is a volatile acid which can dissociate into water and carbon dioxide, the latter being exhaled. A metabolic acidosis occurs when the ratio is altered due to a fall in bicarbonate because of a loss of ions from the body or an accumulation of fixed acids which release hydrogen ions. An example here is low cardiac output states, when cellular hypoxia results in anaerobic metabolism with the release of lactic acid.

Conversely, a respiratory alkalosis is reflected in a fall in $PaCO_2$ due to hyperventilation. In a metabolic alkalosis there is an increase in HCO_3^- due to either excessive alkali intake or a net loss of hydrogen ions from the body, e.g. vomiting/nasogastric aspiration and excessive diuresis. Table 3.3 outlines the main causes of both respiratory and metabolic acid–base abnormalities. Sometimes both acidosis and alkalosis will be present at the same time. One will be causing the primary problem and the other will be an attempt, successful or otherwise, at secondary compensation. Similarly, both respiratory and metabolic acidosis can coexist in disorders such as cardiorespiratory arrest, chronic obstructive pulmonary disease complicated by heart failure, severe pulmonary oedema, and combined respiratory and renal failure.

Several compensatory mechanisms are activated in the body to restore acid–base balance:

- The buffer system is activated almost immediately and involves bicarbonate, proteins and phosphates accepting hydrogen ions
- Changes in ventilatory pattern will occur to either remove carbon dioxide (in acidosis) or retain carbon dioxide (in alkalosis)
- The renal system is efficient in either secreting or retaining ions such as bicarbonate and hydrogen. This compensatory mechanism, however, occurs over several days and acute respiratory acidosis can be life threatening

As outlined earlier, tissue oxygenation depends not only upon pulmonary factors but also upon an effective cardiac output. The following section outlines how this is achieved.

Table 3.3   Major causes of acid–base abnormalities following surgery

Abnormality	Causes
Respiratory problem	
Acidosis – increase in $PaCO_2$	Respiratory depression associated with:
	• pain
↑ hydrogen ions	• excessive sedation
↓ pH	• early weaning from ventilation
	Pulmonary compromise due to surgery
	Chronic obstructive pulmonary disease
	Acute asthma
	Acute respiratory infection
Alkalosis – decrease in $PaCO_2$	Hyperventilation, e.g. anxiety
	Early phase of pulmonary compromise where
↓ hydrogen ions	ventilatory drive ↑
↑ pH	
Metabolic problem	
Acidosis – decrease in HCO_3^-	Anaerobic metabolism as a result of poor tissue
	oxygenation
↑ hydrogen ions	Ketoacidosis
↓ pH	Renal disease
increase in fixed acids, e.g. lactic acid	
or	
loss of HCO_3^-	
Alkalosis – increase in HCO_3^-	Vomiting
	Nasogastric aspiration
↓ hydrogen ions	Alkali intake
↑ pH	

Cardiac physiology

Macrostructure of the heart

The heart, sitting within the thoracic cage, comprises a right and left pump, each of which have two chambers. The atria are weaker pumps, moving blood towards the ventricles while the ventricles supply the force that pumps blood around the pulmonary or systemic circulations. Ensuring blood flows in one direction through these chambers are the semilunar, and atrioventricular valves (AV).

Semilunar valves

The semilunar valves lie at the opening of the ventricles; the pulmonary valve at the junction of the right ventricle and pulmonary artery, and the aortic valve where the aorta leaves the left ventricle. These prevent the backflow of blood from the arteries during diastole. In an adult the aortic valve has an opening of approximately 2.5–3.5 cm^2 and is a tri-leaflet structure. The coronary ostia, where the coronary arteries originate, is approximately 1–2 cm above the aortic valve, in the region of the aortic root. The significance of this close proximity to the valve is seen when aortic stenosis results in a decrease in the coronary blood flow and angina. Similar in size to the aortic valve, the pulmonary valve guards the outlet of the right ventricle.

Atrioventricular valves

The atrioventricular valves prevent the backflow of blood from the ventricles to the atria during ventricular contraction. Between the right atria and ventricle sits the tricuspid valve. This has an opening of approximately 4–6 cm^2, and as its name implies, has three cusps. The mitral valve, opening to 2–4 cm^2, lies between the left atria and ventricle, in close proximity to the aortic valve. It is a bi-leaflet structure, with an anterior and posterior cusp. The anterior cusp generally opens and closes to allow the free flow of blood whereas the posterior cusp is relatively immobile. Chordae tendinae are fan-like structures between the atrioventricular valves and the papillary muscle on the heart wall and prevent the closed valve bulging into the atria during ventricular contraction. The papillary muscle contracts, the chordae tendinae tighten and the valve consequently shuts.

The coronary arteries

There are two main coronary arteries: the right and left coronary artery. The left coronary artery rapidly divides into the circumflex and left anterior descending artery. These arteries form further branches that extend over the epicardial surface of the heart and penetrate deep within the endocardium, thereby ensuring the myocardium receives a plentiful blood supply. The arteries become arterioles and capillaries and blood returns to the heart through the coronary veins. The veins follow the same course as the arteries finally feeding into the great cardiac vein and then the coronary sinus that empties into the right atrium (Fig. 3.9). Additional vessels such as the thebesian veins also empty directly into the heart chambers.

Blood flow though the coronary arteries is regulated by local vasodilation in response to need. For example, when the heart muscle has an increased demand for oxygen and nutrients, due possibly to exercise or an acute illness, the coronary arteries are able to dilate up to five-fold. The exact mechanisms involved in this are unclear, although there is general agreement that vasoactive substances are secreted from the endothelial lining of the arteries. These substances, initially identified as endothelial-derived relaxing factor (EDRF), include prostacyclins and nitric oxide which cause the coronary arteries to vasodilate. It is important to note, however, that these substances are only secreted by an intact endothelium. Hence in the presence of coronary heart disease, where atheroma disrupts the endothelium, these factors are not secreted. Instead a vasoconstricting substance or endothelial-derived constricting factor (EDCF) such as prostanoid or endothelin causes vasoconstriction (Levick 2000). Adenosine, although not secreted from the endothelium, is also thought to play a vital role in vasodilation of the

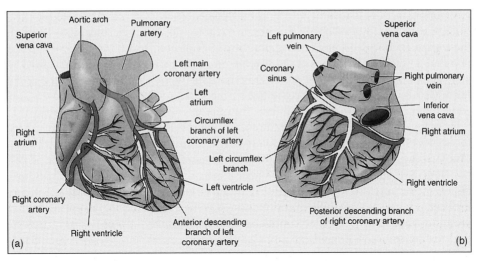

Fig. 3.9 Coronary blood supply. (a) Anterior surface of the heart. (b) Posterior surface of the heart. From Hatchett & Thompson (2002), with permission.

coronary arteries (Ganong 2001) and consequently used in their evaluation (see Chapter 4).

Microstructure of the heart

A cardiac muscle fibre is made up of several individual cells. These long, narrow cells enable the rapid and effective contraction and relaxation of the heart. Figure 3.10 depicts the important features of the cardiac cell. Surrounding the cell is the sarcolemma, or cell membrane, a bi-layer of phospholipid. Within this are various channels, intercalated discs and tubules that enable the rapid movement of ions and electrical charge that results in rapid and coordinated contraction.

The intercalated discs or nexus, form junctions between adjacent cells where they decrease electrical resistance. These communicating gaps are also referred to as gap

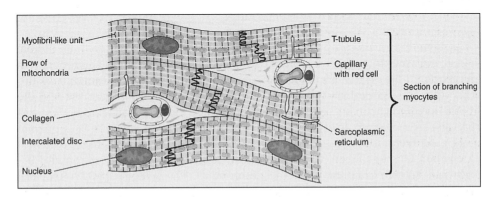

Fig. 3.10 Important features of a cardiac cell. From Hatchett & Thompson (2002), with permission.

junctions (Smith & Kampine 1990). Their permeability is affected by various phy-siological factors. For example, ischaemia is thought to alter permeability through these gap junctions and so decrease myocardial contractility. The transverse tubules (T-tubules) are invaginations of the sarcolemma that cause the extracellular fluid to be in close proximity with the cell interior, furthering the rapid exchange of ions. In other words, the T-tubules increase the surface area of the sarcolemma to the sar-coplasm or cell interior and so enhance the effectiveness of the heart contraction. T-tubules appear to be more developed in the cardiac cell (Guyton & Hall 1996) where the extracellular calcium concentration is important for cardiac cell contraction. Conversely, the sarcoplasmic reticulum is less well developed in the cardiac cell (Downey & Heusch 2001) yet is the major store of intracellular calcium. Therefore, although the calcium ion concentration within the sarcoplasmic reticulum of ske-letal cells influences the force of contraction, it is the extracellular concentration that plays a greater part in cardiac contraction. Approximately 70% of calcium used by the cardiac cell comes from the extracellular fluid. However, the increase in free calcium within the sarcoplasm causes the sarcoplasmic reticulum to release its calcium content that then contributes towards contraction.

Mitochondria are the storehouse for adenosine triphosphate (ATP) and so are important features for cellular function. The great number of mitochondria found in cardiac cells provides a plentiful energy source for the cell and reduces the likelihood of anaerobic cellular metabolism during periods of small oxygen debt (Smith & Kampine 1990). The cardiac cell cannot tolerate oxygen debt, as is seen in myocardial infarction.

Myofibrils

Myofibrils are the contractile portion of the cell. They are rod-like structures that lie longitudinally within the cell and comprise many units, called the sarcomeres. Within each sarcomere are myosin (thick) and actin (thin) filaments. These also lie longitudinally, overlapping to a variable degree. The myosin filaments comprise several myosin molecules. The molecule 'tails' are grouped to form the filament, whereas the 'head' protrudes from the other end. The heads spiral around the length of the filament and it is at this head that ATP is broken down to enable the myosin and actin filaments to interact. Figure 3.11 shows the arrangement of these myofibrils and the cross-bridge formation.

The actin filaments comprise bead-like protein molecules arranged in a double strand of filaments that spiral around themselves. Two other proteins, tropomysin and troponin, lie on this filament and regulate the interaction of the myosin and actin filaments. When the cell is relaxed, troponin and tropomysin prevent the interaction of the actin and myosin filaments. When the electrical charge of the cell changes, free calcium ions bind with the troponin molecule. The tropomysin molecules move, utilising energy, and the filaments are able to loosely attach to each other. Once attached, the myosin head performs a 'rowing' action and the actin and myosin filaments slide over each other. The actin head then detaches itself and reattaches to another myosin molecule to 'row' again. This occurs possibly 40 times during the course of one contraction and demonstrates the amount of energy utilised with each cardiac cell contraction. This process is

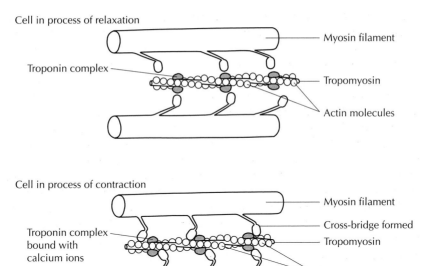

Cell in process of relaxation

Myosin filament

Troponin complex

Tropomyosin

Actin molecules

Cell in process of contraction

Myosin filament

Cross-bridge formed

Troponin complex
bound with
calcium ions

Tropomyosin

Actin molecules

Fig. 3.11 Cross-bridge formation.

referred to as excitation–contraction coupling and results in shortening of the fibre length and muscle contraction.

It is clear, then, that the number of cross-bridges that form influence the force of contraction, or intropic state, and is dependent upon the period of time that calcium is freely available within the cell. As cross-bridges can only form where there is some overlapping of the actin and myosin fibres, the state of stretch of the resting fibre length will also influence the force of contraction. When calcium leaves the cell, the troponin and tropomysin complexes return to their original positions and the heart relaxes. This explains how the administration of intravenous calcium effectively increases the force of cardiac cell contraction while having a lesser effect upon the skeletal muscle cell.

Electrical conduction

Another unique feature of the heart is its ability to initiate and propagate an impulse. The sinus node, situated on the superior lateral wall of the right atrium close to the opening of the vena cava, has its own intrinsic firing rate of 60–100 beats per minute. As this is the fastest rate within the conduction system, the sinus node will normally act as the pacemaker to the heart. From the sinus node, the impulse spreads across the atrium (both right and left) and then to the atrioventricular (AV) node. How the impulse is conducted through the atria is unclear. It is generally considered that there are three internodal tracts: the anterior, middle and posterior internodal pathways. These are small bundles of fibres that enable the propagation of the impulse (Guyton & Hall 1996). Interestingly, there is no histological evidence for these pathways (Thompson 1983; Moorman & Lamers

1999) and it may be that the conduction just passes through atrial tissue to the AV node. Fibrous tissue separates the atria and ventricles and surrounds the opening of the valves. Throughout this tissue are specialised conduction pathways such as the Bundle of His that enable the propagation of the action potential.

Action potential of the cardiac cell

The myocardial cell has specific electrical properties that are dependent upon the difference in electrical charge of the extracellular and intracellular fluid – the potential difference. The ions of particular relevance to this electrical charge are sodium, potassium, calcium and chloride. The interior of the cell is more negatively charged than the extracellular fluid and has a higher concentration of potassium ions (150 mmol/l : 3.5–4.5 mmol/l). This gives the resting ventricular muscle cell, a potential difference of −90 mV. This resting membrane potential is created and maintained by the active transport of potassium ions into the cell, and the outward movement of sodium ions. The higher concentration of potassium ions within the cell, leads to a constant efflux of potassium ions according to their concentration gradient. Therefore this active transport, against a concentration gradient, is essential for efficient cellular function.

Excitation of the cell begins when an electrical stimulus results in an inward current of positively charged ions and the action potential is triggered (see Fig. 3.12). Fast sodium channels within the sarcolemma open and an inward current of positively charged sodium ions rapidly changes the electrical charge from around

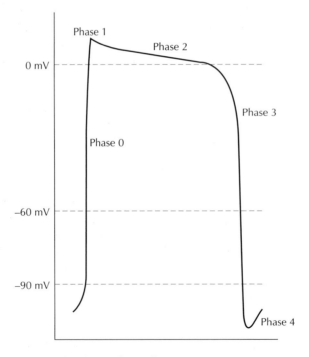

Fig. 3.12 Action potential of the cardiac cell.

−90 mV to +30 mV (phase 0). This rapid depolarisation is best seen in the upstroke of the action potential of the ventricular muscle cells. As it is dependent upon the influx of sodium, extracellular sodium concentration is important. A serum sodium of <140 mmol/l will lead to a reduced upstroke and hence amplitude of the action potential. Once the action potential is triggered, the permeability of the cell wall to potassium ions decreases and potassium is no longer able to move outwards. Also during the latter stages of phase 0, slow calcium and sodium channels open and contribute to the influx of positively charged ions. This is another unique feature of the cardiac cell (Guyton & Hall 1996) and helps to prolong the duration of the action potential. The increase in intracellular calcium also alters the electrical resistance of the gap junctions and potassium does not move out (Smith & Kampine 1990) also contributing towards the plateau phase.

Following the rapid entry of sodium, the fast sodium channels close and the cell voltage starts to fall to around 0 (phase 1). Calcium continues to enter the cell and the sarcoplasmic reticulum releases its calcium content. The electrical charge of the cell is maintained at a constant level and is referred to as the plateau phase (phase 2). It is the uniqueness of this plateau phase that gives a longer duration to the action potential and enables the cardiac muscle cell to contract 3–15 times longer than skeletal muscle (Guyton & Hall 1996; Wahler 2001). The plateau is pronounced still further in the ventricular cells where it is necessary for effective ventricular contraction.

During phase 3, the calcium channels close. Calcium no longer enters the cell and is actively pumped back into the sarcoplasmic reticulum or the extracellular fluid. The efflux of potassium starts again and the cell voltage rapidly moves towards its negative resting voltage. The resting membrane potential (RMP) is then maintained at around −90 mV by the active transport of sodium out of and potassium into the cell. The maintenance of this RMP is referred to as phase 4.

Factors affecting the RMP of the cell will affect the rapid influx of sodium ions, and therefore phase 0 of the action potential. For example, hypokalaemia increases the potential difference and the velocity of depolarisation will therefore increase. It is important to note, however, that when the serum potassium falls below 3 mmol, then the opposite effect occurs (Smith & Kampine 1990). In the same way, if the resting membrane potential becomes less negative, as occurs in hyperkalaemia, the influx of sodium ions takes place through the slow channels and the velocity of depolarisation is reduced.

Throughout the conduction system, the action potential differs. For example, the RMP of the cells of the sinus node are in a constant state of flux. Sodium gradually leaks into the cell causing the voltage to become less negative. An action potential is triggered and the cells spontaneously depolarise (Wahler 2001). More distal to the sinus node, the slope of the RMP is more gradual, leading to the slower intrinsic firing rates of the atrial and ventricular tissue.

Mechanical events of the cardiac cycle

Blood flow through the heart occurs due to pressure changes and gravity. This cycle of events is termed the cardiac cycle. Each cardiac cycle consists of relaxation, or diastole, and a period of contraction or systole, and is depicted in Fig. 3.13.

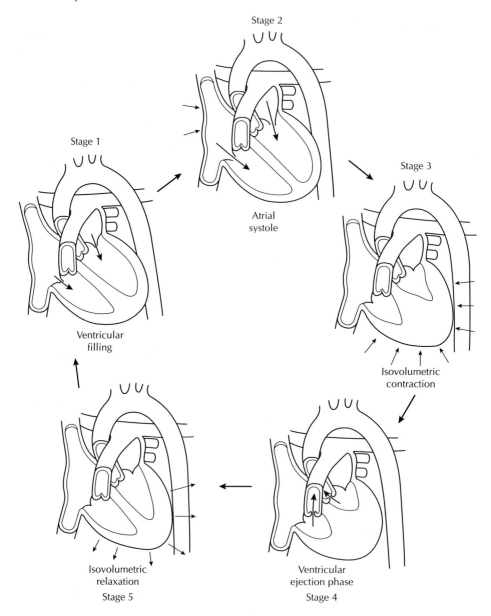

Stage 2

Atrial
systole

Stage 1

Ventricular
filling

Stage 3

Isovolumetric
contraction

Isovolumetric
relaxation
Stage 5

Ventricular
ejection phase
Stage 4

Fig. 3.13   Cardiac cycle.

Blood enters the atria from the inferior and superior vena cavae and pulmonary vein, and then moves passively through an open AV valve into the ventricle. This ventricular filling accounts for 75% of the final ventricular blood volume. When the heart starts to contract, atrial systole occurs forcing the last remaining volume of blood into the ventricles and is sometimes referred to as the 'atrial kick'. These first two stages of the cardiac cycle occur during ventricular diastole and form the diastolic filling time of the heart. When the heart rate increases, this period of diastole is shortened and the volume of blood entering the ventricle consequently decreases. This should not become clinically apparent unless the heart rate exceeds 130 beats per minute (Riley 2002). However, the loss of atrial systole, as occurs in atrial fibrillation, may compromise the haemodynamic status at a slower rate.

The electrical impulse then passes to the AV node, and ventricular contraction starts. The papillary muscles contract to force the AV valves shut and prevent any further movement of blood into the ventricles. The volume of blood in each ventricle at this point is referred to as the end-diastolic volume (EDV) and approximates 120 ml. The ventricle continues to contract in what is termed iso-volumetric contraction, until the pressure within it exceeds the pressure in the pulmonary or systemic circulation and the semilunar valves are forced open and blood is ejected (ventricular ejection). The amount of blood ejected from the ventricle represents about 70% of the total ventricular volume and is known as the stroke volume. In an average adult, this is approximately 80 ml. The volume of blood remaining in the ventricle (end-systolic volume, ESV) is therefore approximately 40 ml. There is considerable variation in the ESV. If the heart contracts more forcibly, the stroke volume may increase and the ESV will consequently decrease. This cardiac reserve, then, is essential to enable the changes in stroke volume associated with the ability to exercise or to cope with increased metabolic demands. Ventricular relaxation then occurs, the semilunar valves snap shut, and the cardiac cycle repeats itself.

The purpose of the cardiac cycle is to create a cardiac output, which is the volume of blood pumped out of the heart in one minute. As the average adult stroke volume is approximately 70 ml, and the heart rate 70 bpm, the cardiac output will be 70 × 70 (4900 ml) or just under 5 litres per minute at rest.

Preload, contractility and afterload

When referring to the cardiac output, three terms are frequently used: preload, contractility and afterload. Variations in these will affect the cardiac output.

Preload
Preload refers to the force that stretches the resting myocardium and so determines the resting length of the sarcomeres. This force is related to the EDV and is closely approximated to the right atrial pressure or pulmonary artery wedge pressure, frequently used as clinical indicators of preload. The preload is therefore a product of ventricular filling and atrial systole and is important in influencing the stroke volume and hence cardiac output. Various factors that may affect the preload are outlined in Table 3.4.

Contractility
Contractility refers to the inotropic state of the heart and the extent and velocity of shortening of the sarcomeres. Through the movement of calcium into the cell, cross-bridges form, and the sarcomere shortens. The force that is generated in this shortening relates to contractility. Contractility is also influenced by the stretch of

Table 3.4 Factors affecting preload

Increased preload	Decreased preload
■ Vasoconstriction ■ Transfusion of blood or fluid ■ Head down position ■ Increased skeletal pumping action; dynamic exercise	■ Vasodilation ■ Hypovolaemia: haemorrhage, dehydration ■ Standing ■ Decreased respiratory pumping action; positive pressure ventilation, raised intrathoracic pressure, Valsalva manoeuvre ■ Cardiac tamponade, constrictive pericarditis ■ Tension pneumothorax ■ Arrhythmias, e.g. atrial fibrillation, atrial flutter, AV dissociation

the sarcomere in its resting state. This stretch increases the number of cross-bridges that are able to form through being in close proximity. However, it may be that the stretch of the resting sarcomere increases its sensitivity to intracellular calcium and so facilitates calcium release from the sarcoplasmic reticulum (Skarvan 2000). Levick (2000) suggests that the increased sensitivity may be facilitated through stretch-sensitive channels in the sarcolemma that respond to the increased fibre length and so increase intracellular calcium. Either way, the increase in intracellular calcium enables a greater number of cross-bridges to form, detach and reattach, and improves sliding of the filaments and shortening of the muscle length.

This inotropic state of the heart can be increased though endogenous and exogenous sources (see Table 3.5). Previously the role of intravenous calcium has been discussed in relation to how it can increase the force of contraction of the heart and so act as an exogenous inotrope. Similarly, catecholamines, whether naturally occurring as part of the stress response or administered pharmacologically as epinephrine, increase intracellular calcium and hence the force of contraction. Digoxin also has an inotropic action, and by binding with the sodium and potassium pumps prevents sodium being extruded from the cell. Intracellular sodium concentration consequently increases. This in turn activates the sodium/calcium exchange pump. Sodium is expelled from the cell in exchange for calcium

Table 3.5 Factors affecting contractility

Increased contractility	Decreased contractility
■ Sympathetic nervous system stimulation ■ Catecholamines, exogenous and endogenous ■ Angiotensin II ■ Intravenous calcium ■ Increased myocardial oxygen delivery ■ Increased preload	■ Myocardial hypoxia ■ Pharmacological depressants: beta blockers, calcium channel blockers, most anaesthetic agents ■ Metabolic depressants; acidosis ■ Decreased preload ■ Increased afterload

and the intracellular concentration of calcium rises. The consequence is an increase in free calcium and an increase in contractility.

Afterload

Afterload describes the force that opposes the shortening of the sarcomeres and hence contraction of the ventricles. It is determined by the impedance to flow and ventricular wall tension. Wall tension, determined by the law of Laplace, states the relationship between the radius of the chamber, its pressure and thickness. Hence, afterload depends upon the radius of the ventricle as well as the ejection pressure. As the volume or radius increases, so the afterload will also increase. Therefore, as the ventricle ejects blood, the radius reduces and there is a gradual reduction in afterload, making the latter stages of ventricular ejection easier.

Contractility is inversely related to afterload. Therefore, an increase in afterload will decrease the extent and velocity of sarcomere shortening (see Table 3.6).

Table 3.6 Factors affecting afterload

Increased afterload	Decreased afterload
■ Increased aortic impedance	■ Decreased aortic impedance
■ Aortic stenosis	■ Arteriolar dilation
■ Vasoconstriction	■ Reduced ventricular cavity size
■ Dilation of ventricular cavity	

The relevance and interrelationships between the three terms is seen through the Frank–Starling law of cardiac contractility (Fig. 3.14). This law states that there is a relationship between the length of the muscle filament and the tension generated. In other words, as the filaments are stretched, greater tension is generated and the ensuing force of contraction (velocity) will be greater. A greater volume of blood will then be pumped out of the ventricle. If the muscle

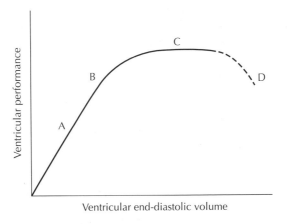

Fig. 3.14 Frank–Starling law of cardiac contractility.

cells are insufficiently stretched, shortening will be less and the force of contraction, reduced. Therefore the amount of blood in the resting ventricle, the preload, will influence the amount of stretch on the muscle cells, and hence the stroke volume.

Curve A on Fig. 3.14 demonstrates this linear relationship: as the preload increases, stroke volume will also increase. Similarly, if available calcium is increased, as occurs at greater fibre length, the inotropic state of the heart will increase the stroke volume still further. This is depicted on the latter part of this curve at point B. The correlation between the end-diastolic volume and tension is not always linear, and this is represented in the plateau phase of the curve C. Here, an increase in preload will not increase the stroke volume. Applying the law of Laplace, we can see how an increase in preload will also increase afterload and impede ventricular output. In health, the increased contractile force overrides this potentially negative effect. However, in the failing heart, the increase in afterload created by the increased preload seriously impairs the heart's pumping action and leads to a reduced cardiac output, shown as point D on the curve.

In the short-term, an increase in heart rate appears to increase myocardial contractility, possibly through β-adrenergic stimulation (Skarvan 2000) as well as through increasing preload, and offers benefit. However, a long-term tachycardia appears to have adverse effects. In health, then, it can be seen how the function of the heart is determined by the interplay of preload, afterload and contractility. Ill health changes these relationships and contributes towards a worsening spiral of physiological consequences. Many of our interventions as cardiothoracic surgical nurses aim to influence favourably these factors.

Cardiovascular regulatory mechanisms

Earlier, the role of the lungs and heart in contributing to effective oxygen delivery was outlined. The integrity of the peripheral circulation is also important in this respect and ensures that the oxygenated blood ejected by the left ventricle is delivered and tissue perfusion pressure maintained. Blood pressure (BP) is determined by the cardiac output (CO) and systemic vascular resistance (SVR):

$$BP = CO \times SVR$$

The peripheral circulation is made up of a vast, complex network of blood vessels which can be divided into three main sections:

- **Arterial bed including arterioles:** distributes the cardiac output to the various regions of the body
- **Capillary bed:** perfuses the tissues thus supplying cells with oxygen, nutrients and additional factors
- **Venous system:** returns deoxygenated blood to the heart

Following cardiac and thoracic surgery, haemodynamic changes can occur quickly and can seriously compromise tissue perfusion. When this occurs a number of compensatory mechanisms are activated to preserve effective perfusion pressures so that normal cellular function is maintained.

Systemic arterial system

It is in the smaller arteries and arterioles where most of the resistance to blood flow is found. So important is the vascular resistance of the arterial bed that a number of factors contribute to its control. First of all, stimulation of the sympathetic nervous system results in the release of norepinephrine which targets adrenergic α receptors found on the smooth muscle cell membrane in the tunica media of these vessels. This is mediated through the vasomotor centre in the medulla oblongata which helps to maintain a steady state of contraction of this muscle. The peripheral vessels in the kidney, skin, spleen and mesentery are particularly well supplied with α receptors so that when peripheral resistance needs to be increased this is not at the expense of perfusion to the brain, heart and skeletal muscle. This α receptor activity ensures that blood is diverted to key areas while peripheral resistance and therefore blood pressure is maintained.

Sympathetic nerves supply the adrenal medulla but at this site it is the neurotransmitter acetylcholine which stimulates the release of norepinephrine and epinephrine. Norepinephrine results in α receptor effects (vasoconstriction) and epinephrine results in β receptor effects. Beta effects are mediated through β_2 receptors in skeletal muscle and cardiac blood vessels and result in relaxation and therefore less vasoconstriction. It is the α receptor response via the sympathetic nervous system which is responsible for the 'peripheral shutdown' which occurs in haemodynamically compromised states (cool extremities with pallor and reduced urine output).

Local effects are also responsible for changes to arteriolar resistance. Increase in body heat for example, as in rewarming following cardiac surgery or because of infection, will dilate blood vessels both locally and also through thermoreceptors in the hypothalamus. Through this vasodilatory action heat is quickly lost from the body. Levels of carbon dioxide can increase resistance and high PCO_2 levels can also cause vasodilation with a fall in resistance. Hypoxia can similarly result in constriction of vessels through the sympathetic nervous system and, again, with severe hypoxia this can result in local dilation and reduced vascular resistance. Accumulation of hydrogen ions as a result of acidosis (e.g. lactic acid) can result in vasodilation of resistance vessels (Ganong 2001).

The capillary bed

The capillaries make up the microcirculation and these vessels have thin walls with no smooth muscle. The structure of the capillary is important as although there is only 5% of the blood volume in the capillaries at any one time the semipermeable nature of the capillary walls allows perfusion of the tissues and the removal of waste products. The cross-sectional area of the capillary bed is quite large and blood flow decreases allowing this exchange to take place. At the origin of the capillary there is often a small band of muscle which serves as a precapillary sphincter. Closure of these sphincters allows sections of the capillary bed to be closed off thereby diverting blood to other areas, and at rest many capillaries are closed. When tissues become more metabolically active the following local factors result in relaxation of the pre-capillary sphincter and vasodilation:

- Increase in CO_2
- Fall in PO_2
- Fall in pH

When there is local tissue damage then capillaries may vasodilate in response to agents such as substance P, bradykinin and serotonin. Histamine released by mast cells in response to an allergen will also vasodilate and increase permeability.

Venous circulation

Capillaries drain blood into venules and then larger veins. Vein walls are thinner than those of arteries and vein diameter is greater, allowing distension. Whereas the arteries and arterioles are called resistance vessels the veins are referred to as capacitance vessels because of their ability to act as a reservoir for blood. Venous flow is aided by the increase in negative intrathoracic pressure during inspiration, skeletal muscle contraction which compresses the veins and the presence of valves preventing backflow.

Veins also have a sympathetic nerve supply. When stimulated by norepinephrine muscle tone will increase, the venous bed will constrict and venous return, and therefore preload to the heart, will increase.

Pulmonary circulation

Deoxygenated blood is pumped by the right ventricle into the pulmonary arteries and this blood is referred to as mixed venous blood. Pulmonary arteries eventually branch into pulmonary capillaries, and the pulmonary circulation is responsible for perfusing the lungs thus ensuring that each alveolus has a capillary network for the exchange of oxygen and carbon dioxide.

Approximately 70 ml of blood flows through the pulmonary capillaries at any one time. Compared with the systemic circulation the pulmonary circulation is a high-volume, low-pressure system. The thin walls of the pulmonary arteries contain much less muscle than the systemic arteries and this results in much lower resistance overall. Figure 3.15 compares the pressures within the systemic and pulmonary circulations.

At rest, not all pulmonary capillary networks are open and this results in different ventilation/perfusion relationships throughout the lungs. With an increase in cardiac output, perfusion increases and more capillaries are recruited, facilitating greater gaseous exchange. Pulmonary blood vessels also have neural and hormonal control mechanisms. Sympathetic and parasympathetic nerve fibres result in vasoconstriction and vasodilation respectively. Factors which increase pulmonary vascular resistance include epinephrine, norepinephrine, serotonin, histamine and thromboxane. Conversely, acetylcholine, some prostaglandins and prostacyclin result in pulmonary vasodilation.

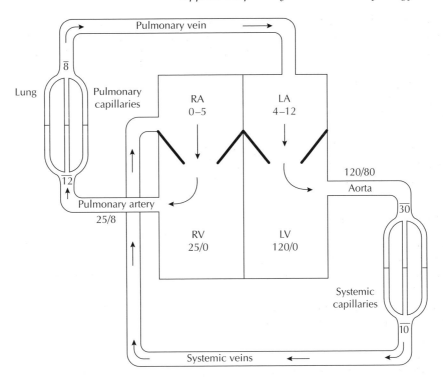

Fig. 3.15 Systemic and pulmonary pressures (mmHg).

Alveolar hypoxia results in localised pulmonary vasoconstriction which diverts the blood towards areas that are better ventilated. This mechanism is referred to as hypoxic pulmonary vasoconstriction. With some pulmonary diseases this response may lead to very high pulmonary pressures due to increased resistance and resulting in right ventricular strain.

Maintenance of blood pressure in the peripheral circulation

A number of compensatory mechanisms are activated when haemodynamic status is altered. Autoregulation is the mechanism whereby local blood flow and oxygen delivery to an organ are maintained. Although it is well developed in the kidneys it is also seen in other tissues such as the myocardium and brain. The metabolic theory explaining this response highlights the importance of vasodilator substances such as lactic acid which accumulates in metabolically active tissues (Ganong 2001). The myogenic theory of autoregulation stresses the contractile response of smooth muscle to tension in the vessel wall and follows the law of Laplace where wall tension is proportional to the distending pressure times the radius.

Many internal organs of the body are innervated by both sympathetic and parasympathetic nerve fibres and their neurotransmitters cause excitation or inhibition depending on the receptor site targeted. A major component of physiological control of blood pressure involves complex sensory signalling by the central nervous system affecting cardiac and vascular targets (Rea & Thames 1993). Increased sympathetic nervous activity is a major component of the compensation which occurs when systemic blood pressure falls. High pressure arterial baroreceptors in the carotid sinus and aortic arch respond to falls in blood pressure by increasing sympathetic discharge from the vasomotor centre in the brain stem. There are also low-pressure baroreceptors in the heart and pulmonary vessels which sense low volume (Feton *et al.* 2000). Overall decrease in sensory output from these baroreceptors ultimately increases sympathetic tone. Once blood pressure increases then a feedback mechanism results in increased baroreceptor firing which increases the parasympathetic/vagal response.

Sympathetic activity results in excitation of α receptors by norepinephrine in peripheral vessels and redirects blood to essential areas increasing vascular resistance and venous return. The resulting vasoconstriction reduces hydrostatic pressure in capillary beds promoting the redistribution of fluid from the extravascular compartment into the capillary lumen (Sielenkamper & Sibbald 2000).

Stimulation of β receptors by sympathetic arousal includes the following effects:

- Cardiac (β_1): increased rate, conduction and contraction
- Coronary arteries (β_2): vasodilation with increased myocardial perfusion
- Respiratory smooth muscle (β_2): relaxation with bronchodilation

In addition to the above, early neural response hormonal mechanisms attempt to further increase the intravascular volume and this is mediated through:

- Renin–angiotensin system
- Antidiuretic hormone (ADH)
- Adrenocorticotrophic hormone (ACTH)

Systemic factors in vasoactive regulation

As well as autoregulatory and neurohormonal responses there are a number of systemic factors which can have a powerful effect on vessels. Table 3.7 gives examples of various agents which demonstrate a vasoactive effect. A major source of many of these vasoactive mediators is endothelial cells.

Figure 3.16 summarises the compensatory changes which occur following haemorrhage. However, there are a number of disorders resulting in hypotension, and although the eventual outcome will be the same if left untreated in terms of cellular ischaemia and death, the underlying mechanisms resulting in compromise vary. Because the maintenance of an adequate cardiac output is a key determinant of systemic blood pressure, circulatory support will invariably involve manipulation of preload, myocardial contractility, afterload and heart rate (Hinds & Watson 1999).

This chapter has explored the physiological mechanisms which contribute towards effective tissue oxygenation. Awareness by the nurse of these physiological mechanisms and responses will not only aid in guiding patient assessment but also increase understanding of the rationale underpinning the myriad of

Table 3.7   Examples of vasoactive agents

Factor	Source	Blood vessels	Additional effects
Nitric oxide (NO)	Epithelial cells Endothelial cells NANC nerves	Vasodilator	Bronchodilator
Vasoactive intestinal polypeptide (VIP)	NANC nerves	Vasodilator	Bronchodilator
Histamine	Mast cells	Vasodilator	Bronchoconstrictor
Prostaglandins: PGI_2 PGE_1	Arachidonic acid in cell membranes	Vasodilators	
PGH_2 $PGF_2\alpha$	Arachidonic acid in cell membrane	Vasoconstrictors	Bronchoconstrictors
Kinins: Bradykinin Kalidin	Tissue cells Plasma	Vasodilator	Contracts visceral smooth muscle Increases capillary permeability
Prostacyclin	Endothelial cells	Vasodilator	Inhibits platelet aggregation
Thromboxane A_2	Arachidonic acid in cell membranes (e.g. endothelial cells and platelets)	Vasoconstrictor	Platelet aggregation
Angiotensin II	Renin–angiotensin	Vasoconstrictor	
Endothelin I	Endothelial cells	Potent vasoconstrictor	Bronchoconstrictor cardiac contraction ↑ heart rate ↑ renal blood flow ↑

therapeutic interventions. Figure 3.17 gives a useful overview of the many factors to consider in ensuring that oxygen supply keeps up with oxygen demand.

Hypotension, which is not reversed, can result not only in direct cellular damage but also in the initiation of a complex systemic inflammatory response leading to further perfusion problems and widespread tissue injury (Waxman 1996). If oxygen delivery is not optimised then maintenance of cellular function is not possible, and if cellular ischaemia is not corrected then organ failure and death are inevitable consequences (Shoemaker *et al.* 1992). Haemodynamic instability can develop at any time in the post-operative period although it is more common in the first 24–48 hours. A sound knowledge of pulmonary and cardiovascular regulatory mechanisms will assist in the early recognition of problems and in the timely utilisation of effective strategies.

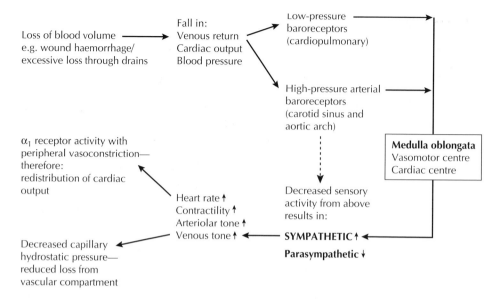

Fig. 3.16 Compensatory changes following haemorrhage.

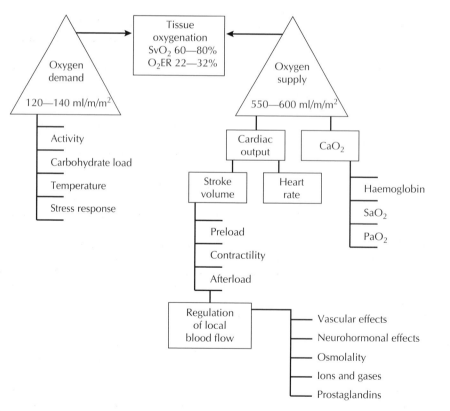

Fig. 3.17 Determinants of tissue oxygenation. From Jesurum (1997), with permission.

References

Al-Ali, M.K. & Howarth, P.H. (1998) Nitric oxide and the respiratory system in health and disease. *Respiratory Medicine* **92**: 701–15.

Barnes, P.J. (1986) Neural control of human airways in health and disease. *American Review of Respiratory Disease* **134**: 1289–1314.

Barnes, P.J., Baranuik, J.N. & Belvisi, M.G. (1991) Neuropeptides in the respiratory tract: part 1. *American Review of Respiratory Disease* **144**: 1187–9.

Beachey, W. (1998) *Respiratory Care Anatomy and Physiology: Foundations for Clinical Practice.* Mosby, London.

Belvisi, M.G., Stretton, C.D. & Barnes, P.J. (1992) Nitric oxide is the endogenous neurotransmitter of bronchodilator nerves in human airways. *European Journal of Pharmacology* **210**: 221–2.

Brismar, B., Hedenstierna, G., Lundquist, H, *et al.* (1985) Pulmonary densities during anaesthesia with muscular relaxation – a proposal for atelectasis. *Anaesthesiology* **62**: 422.

D'Oliveira, M., Sykes, M.K., Chakrabarti, M.K., Orchard, C. & Keslin, J. (1981) Depression of hypoxic pulmonary vasoconstriction by sodium nitroprusside and nitroglycerine. *British Journal of Anaesthesiology* **53**: 11–17.

Downey, J. & Heusch, G. (2001) Sequence of cardiac activation and ventricular mechanics. In: Sperelakis, N., Kurachi, Y., Terzix, A. & Cohen, M. (eds) *Heart Physiology and Pathophysiology,* 4th edn. Academic Press, New York.

Feton, A.M., Hammill, S.C., Rea, R.F., Low, P.A. & Shen, W.K. (2000) Vasovagal syncope. *Annals of Internal Medicine* **133**(9): 714–25.

Ganong, W. (2001) *Review of Medical Physiology,* 20th edn. McGraw-Hill, New York.

Guyton, A. & Hall, J. (1996) *Textbook of Medical Physiology,* 9th edn. W.B. Saunders, London.

Hatchett, R. & Thompson, D. (2002) *Cardiac Nursing: A Comprehensive Guide.* Churchill Livingstone, Edinburgh.

Hinds, C.J. & Watson, D. (1999) ABC of intensive care: circulatory support. *British Medical Journal* **318**(7200): 1749–52.

Jesurum, J. (1997) Tissue oxygenation and routine nursing procedures in critically ill patients. *Journal of Cardiovascular Nursing* **11**(4): 12–29.

Joos, G.F., Germonpre, P.R. & Pauwels, R.A. (1995) Neurogenic inflammation in human airways: is it important? *Thorax* **50**: 217–19.

Levick, J.R. (2000) *An Introduction to Cardiovascular Physiology,* 3rd edn. Arnold, London.

Moorman, A. & Lamers, W. (1999) Development of the conduction system of the vertebrate heart. In: Harvey, R. & Rosenthal, H. (eds) *Heart Development.* Academic Press, San Diego, CA.

Mynster, T., Jensen, L.M., Jensen, F.G., Kehlet, H. & Rosenberg, J. (1996) The effect of posture on late postoperative hypoxaemia. *Anaesthesia* **51**: 225–7.

Nomoto, Y. & Kawamura, M. (1989) Pulmonary gas exchange effects by nitroglycerine, dopamine and dobutamine during one lung ventilation in man. *Canadian Journal of Anaesthesia* **36**: 273–7.

Rea, R.F. & Thames, M.D. (1993) Neural control mechanisms and vasovagal syncope. *Journal of Cardiovascular Electrophysiology* **4**: 587–95.

Rennotte, M.T., Reynaert, M., Clerbaux., TH. *et al.* (1989) The effects of two inotropic drugs, dopamine and dobutamine on pulmonary gas exchange in artificially ventilated patients. *Intensive Care Medicine* **15**: 160–65.

Riley, J. (2002) The ECG: its role and practical application. In: Hatchett, R. & Thompson, D. (eds) *Cardiac Nursing: A Comprehensive Guide.* Churchill Livingstone, Edinburgh.

Sadeghi Hashjin, G., Folkerts, G., Henricks, P.A. *et al.* (1996) Peroxynitrite induces airway hyperresponsiveness in guinea pigs in vitro and in vivo. *American Journal of Respiratory and Critical Care Medicine* **153**: 1687–701.

Savov, J. (1995) Surfactant system of the lung: historical perspective. *Seminars in Respiratory Critical Care Medicine* **16**(1): 1.

Shoemaker, W.C., Appel, P.L. & Kram, H.B. (1992) Role of oxygen debt in the development of organ failure sepsis, and death in the high risk surgical patients. *Chest* **102**: 108–15.

Sielenkamper, A. & Sibbald, W.J. (2000) Pathophysiology of hypotension In: Webb, A.R. *et al.* (eds) *Oxford Textbook of Critical Care.* Oxford University Press, Oxford.

Skarvan, K. (2000) Ventricular performance In: Priebe, H. & Skevan, K. (eds) *Cardiovascular Physiology,* 2nd edn. BMJ Publishing Group, London.

Slutsky, A.S. & Tremblay, L.N. (1998) Multiple organ failure. Is mechanical ventilation a contributing factor? *American Journal of Respiratory Critical Care Medicine* **157**(6 Pt 1): 1721–5.

Smith, J. & Kampine, J. (1990) *Circulatory Physiology – The Essentials,* 3rd edn. Williams & Wilkins, Baltimore.

Spina, D. (1996) Airway sensory nerves: a burning issue is asthma? *Thorax* **51**(3): 335–7.

Thompson, D. (1983) Specialized internodal pathways. *International Journal of Cardiology* **4**: 393–6.

Wahler, G. (2001) Cardiac action potential. In: Sperelakis, N., Kurachi, Y., Terzix, A. & Cohen, M. (eds) *Heart Physiology and Pathophysiology,* 4th edn. Academic Press, New York.

Waxman, K. (1996) Shock: ischaemia, reperfusion and inflammation. *New Horizons* **4**: 153–60.

Weibel, E.R. (1963) *Morphometry of the Human Lung.* Springer-Verlag, Berlin.

Widdicombe, J. & Davies, A. (1983) *Respiratory Physiology.* Edward Arnold, London.

4
Pre-operative Preparation

For a small group of patients, surgery will be an unexpected event and the opportunity for a full assessment will not be possible. For most, however, surgery is elective and time will be available for the nurse to carry out the assessment, an important objective being to prepare the patient both physically and psychologically for surgery. Patients awaiting surgery frequently experience not only worsening symptoms such as increasing breathlessness, chest pain and immobility, but also anxiety and fear (Billing *et al.* 1996; Doogue *et al.* 1997; Fitzsimons *et al.* 2000). Common fears relate to not waking from the anaesthesia, being diagnosed with cancer, suffering pain after surgery, and absence from home or work (Bengston *et al.* 1996; Mark *et al.* 1997). Heightened anxiety and fear may be associated with poorer outcome including longer hospital stays, delayed wound healing and higher rates of rehospitalisation (Kiecolt-Glaser *et al.* 1998).

For the person awaiting cardiothoracic surgery, anxieties may be compounded by the serious nature of heart surgery, the extent of any tumour, or fear that they may have to wait too long for the operation. Indeed, waiting is frequently lengthy and it is during this period that appropriate nursing intervention can help towards ensuring that maximum benefit is gained from surgery. This chapter reviews the effects of the stress response to surgery while considering the nursing assessment and management that may favourably influence the physiological and psychological status of the patient. While acknowledging the multi-professional nature of health care, this chapter focuses on those issues that are important for the nurse.

The stress response

It has been acknowledged for some time that admission into hospital increases levels of anxiety and stress. Although the stress response is considered adaptive, presenting the individual with an opportunity to master new skills, such a physiological response may be maladaptive, taxing further the reserves of a cardiopulmonary system already compromised. The stress response is mediated through the autonomic nervous system and hypothalamic–pituitary–adrenal axis (HPA). Hans Selye (1956) called this response the general adaptation syndrome (GAS). The principal mediators involved are catecholamines and cortisol acting either as neurotransmitters, hormones or both. Sympathetic arousal with increases in epinephrine and norepinephrine enables the body to cope with increased demands. Oxygen and glucose delivery to the cells are increased to support increased energy expenditure.

Hospitalisation for cardiothoracic surgery, whether elective or emergency, represents a crisis in the person's life. The physical 'trauma' of surgery itself will result in a massive physiological stress response, yet in the absence of this response the maintenance of homeostasis would be impossible and surgical outcome most likely poor. Although the mechanisms involved in psychological stress and surgical stress are very different, both responses will be reviewed when considering pre-operative factors which might increase post-operative risk. There is recognition that, just like the general adaptation syndrome, the surgical stress response is also adaptive, representing a universally conserved cellular defence mechanism (Minowada & Welch 1995). For example, during acute stress under the influence of cortisol, lymphocytes and macrophages are redistributed throughout the body and 'marginate' on blood vessel walls and within certain compartments such as the skin, lymph nodes and bone marrow (Dhabhar *et al.* 1994). This response is important as far as the healing process is concerned and differs from that in chronic stress where there may be a reduction of lymphocytes. Cortisol also contributes to the integrity of the vascular compartment and the circulation generally, and without cortisol circulatory collapse rapidly ensues (Lamberts *et al.* 1997). It has also been suggested that relative adrenal insufficiency resulting in low cortisol may contribute to a fatal outcome, especially in patients with multi-organ failure. Generally, the acute stress response maintains a hypermetabolic state in the peri-operative period, orchestrated by neuroendocrine, metabolic and immune systems. This metabolic activity promotes wound healing and optimises host defences in the peri-operative period.

Knowledge of the possible harmful effects of the stress response during surgery has grown enormously. The pathophysiological changes involved in surgical stress are complex, but in the high-risk patient can contribute to multiple organ dysfunction due to increased demand and difficulties in microcirculatory blood flow, resulting in tissue damage and cell death. Improved mapping techniques have enabled researchers to focus more on the cellular and humoral components of the stress response. A variety of pro-inflammatory mediators are involved including cytokines, nitric oxide and metabolites of arachidonic acid (e.g. prostaglandin PGE_2) released from cell membranes. Cytokines are chemical 'messengers' released by many different cells which enable communication between different cells. Although the HPA axis and sympathetic systems respond to circadian, neural and blood-borne signals, they are also activated by cytokines produced by immune-mediated inflammatory reactions, such as tumour necrosis factor (TNF), interleukin-1 (IL-1) and interleukin-6 (IL-6) (Chrousos & Gold 1992; Papanicolaou *et al.* 1998). By targeting some of these pro-inflammatory agents it may be possible to modify the stress response thus avoiding some of the less desirable aspects.

One effect of surgery under general anaesthetic, and as a result of the stress response, is the depression in cellular and humoral immunity, particularly natural killer cells. The latter are specialised lymphocytes which are cytotoxic to a variety of tumour cells. Major surgery results in a greater increase in corticotrophin-releasing hormone and glucocorticoids from the adrenal cortex. The more invasive the procedure the greater the stress response will be. Such an effect has been demonstrated in patients undergoing open heart surgery (Ryhanen *et al.* 1984) and in surgery for resection of various tumours (Pollock *et al.* 1992). In surgery for malignant tumours, surgeons have experienced difficulty in successfully eliminating a patient's tumour because of this immunosuppression and the development of micro-metastases (Colacchio *et al.* 1994, Craig *et al.* 2001). The consequences of such immunosuppression for the surgical patient in terms of impaired wound healing and infection means that everything possible should be done to attenuate the stress response. Preparation of patients for surgery may increasingly involve the peri-operative maximisation of the immune response in order to improve short-term morbidity and longer-term survival, particularly in patients with cancer (Koltun *et al.* 1996).

Modification of the stress response in the peri-operative period and the achievement of adequate tissue perfusion have become important goals in management (Pollock *et al.* 2000). Although a variety of different approaches have been taken, the definitive therapy is still elusive. The use of pharmaceutical agents which prevent the release of pro-inflammatory agents such as IL-1, IL-6 and TNF would be useful, but to date only glucocorticoids have been studied in elective surgical procedures. Any attempt to modify the inflammatory response during surgery must be made with caution owing to the possible side-effects of immunosuppression. Given the complexities of the altered physiology in surgical stress and its devastating consequences, most would agree that minimal intervention is best. There is an increasing trend in the use of minimally invasive surgery, which reduces the extent of surgical stress and therefore immunosuppression and risk of infection.

Even with the surgical stress response reduced, what of the stress resulting because of psychological factors? As well as the physical trauma of surgery, psychological factors both before and following surgery may also result in significant neurohormonal changes which may not always be adaptive. Emotions and cognitions are powerful triggers of the stress response. The prospect of major surgery for the patient is associated with anxiety and the apprehension of personal injury (Kirschbaum & Hellhammer 1994; Smyth *et al.* 1998). In a study of patients who had undergone coronary angioplasty, high self-esteem, a sense of personal control and an optimistic outlook were linked with positive adjustment following discharge (Helgeson 1999). Feelings of vulnerability together with increased powerlessness, where there is perceived lack of control over the current situation, results in the release of corticotrophin-releasing hormone (CRH) and adrenocorticotrophic hormone (ACTH) with a subsequent rise in cortisol levels (Peters *et al.* 1998). In one study of patients having cardiac surgery, pre-operative salivary cortisol levels increased from 4.1 nmol/l to 39.4 nmol/l, with plasma cortisol levels reaching 419.0 nmol/l before induction of anaesthesia (Bergmann *et al.* 2000). Cortisol levels fell during surgery then rose again post-operatively. This pattern of cortisol secretion has been found in earlier studies of cardiac surgical patients (Tonnesen *et al.* 1987; Hahnel *et al.* 1994). Furthermore, negative emotions can directly affect the cells of the immune system and can cause either an increase or a decrease in the secretion of pro-inflammatory cytokines (Kiecolt-Glaser *et al.* 2002).

Although surgery may follow the sudden onset of symptoms, for many admitted for cardiac or thoracic surgery there has often been a period of trying to cope with a disorder which is chronic in nature with worsening symptoms, increased disability and poor quality of life. Chronic illness presents the individual with a number of challenges which can result in ongoing psychosocial stress. There is increasing evidence of the negative impact of stress on immune function in terms of increased risk of infection and prolonged illness episodes. In one study, middle-aged healthy adults who reported high levels of chronic stress showed suppressed cardiovascular and neuroendocrine responses during acute stress and recovery (Matthews *et al.* 2001). A suggestion here is that with repeated efforts to cope, fatigue develops and the capacity to meet new challenges is depleted. The implications of these findings for surgical patients needs further testing. It may be that the additive effects of the acute stress of surgery, on top of background chronic stress in some patients, may increase risk significantly.

Given that the stress response, while adaptive, can also result in problems for the patient, what measures might be taken in the pre-operative period to minimise any deleterious effects? The skilled nurse is able to draw on a range of appropriate interventions to reduce psychological stress and to contribute towards minimising the effects of the surgical stress response.

No matter how minimally invasive surgery becomes, most patients will continue to perceive such procedures as stressful. Yet if some neuroendocrine activation is inevitable because of the surgical procedure alone, are active measures to reduce psychological stress in the pre-operative period going to affect patient outcome to any significant degree? Is there any evidence to suggest that ongoing anxiety and stress following cardiothoracic surgery has a negative effect on patient outcome? Levels of stress and anxiety can be high following cardiac events such as acute myocardial infarction and coronary artery bypass surgery. Affective difficulties following such events can result in problems with longer-term adjustment including return to work. Unfortunately, few studies have involved patients undergoing thoracic surgery and this is an area where further investigation is urgently needed. Outcome is likely to be affected not only by the type of surgery performed but also by the reasons for surgery in the first place. Patient expectations are important too. Surgery may be seen as a possible cure, yet perceived continuing deterioration and recurrence of symptoms post-operatively for some patients may result in profound disappointment and contribute to feelings of depression. Ongoing support is crucial for patients during this period.

The paradox whereby the stress response can be both protective and yet possibly damaging has been recognised for some time. There is, of course, enormous individual variability in the stress response. Genetic factors account for some of the individual variability but also important is the perception of the individual and a person's state of physical health, determined not only by genetics but also by behavioural and lifestyle choices (McEwen 1998). This paradox is not merely academic but has important practical implications for the patient undergoing cardiothoracic surgery.

To what extent personality, behaviour, coping style and emotional state affect surgical outcome is difficult to say as few studies have been carried out in this area. Although there has been much nursing research looking at the potential benefits of giving information before surgery, less is known about the usefulness of specific psychological interventions. Although studies in psychoneuro-immunology have shown some benefit from psychological interventions, not all studies are conclusive, mainly owing to conceptual and methodological difficulties. Given that emotions can indeed result in changes in immune functioning, there are exciting research opportunities in cardiothoracic surgical nursing exploring the possible benefits of various psychological interventions.

The pre-admission clinic

The pre-admission clinic is gaining popularity and is useful in ensuring both physiological and psychological preparation of the patient and their family. Laboratory blood work can be analysed and treatment commenced prior to hospital admission, breathing exercises can be taught and information given to allay anxieties. In addition, discharge planning can be commenced at this early stage. For example, in the patient with co-morbidities such as angina, peripheral vascular disease or disability, particularly where there is poor social support, a period of convalescence can be organised well in advance of hospital discharge.

As early as the 1960s the importance of pre-operative information in reducing pain was demonstrated (Egbert *et al.* 1964). A little later the seminal works of Boore (1978) Hayward (1975) and Wilson-Barnett (1979) endorsed the association between pre-operative information and reduced levels of anxiety, pain and shorter hospital stay, suggesting that patient satisfaction would improve as people were given an opportunity to discuss their anxieties and become familiar with the surgical procedure.

Information-seeking coping strategies are used by patients predominately during the pre-operative period and pre-operative information, given either the day of hospital admission or during a pre-operative clinic visit, has become standard practice (King 1985). Interestingly, recent studies do not support this

(MacPherson & Lofgren 1994), and patients are often dissatisfied with the information they are given pre-operatively (Davenport 1991; Bengston *et al.* 1996). A recent large randomised controlled trial investigating the impact of pre-operative education on post-operative anxiety failed to show any significant difference between the groups in levels of anxiety, pain, depression or well-being (Shuldham 1999). The lack of consensus in these findings warrants further discussion and may possibly result from changes in patients' expectations regarding the outcome of their surgery or may allude to the timing and content of the information. The question that remains, therefore, surrounds not so much the benefit or otherwise of pre-operative information as the appropriate use of education strategies regarding content, delivery and timing.

Immediately prior to major surgery it is not surprising to discover that the patient is very anxious (Fitzsimons *et al.* 2000), and although learning may be increased by anxiety, too much anxiety may create a negative effect and impair their capacity to retain further information. In two small-scale studies, patients were less anxious between 5 and 14 days prior to hospital admission (Cupples 1991; Klopfenstein *et al.* 2000). Consequently, information given during this time may be more effectively retained. However, this is not widely agreed and others have suggested that information given 1–3 weeks prior to surgery may exacerbate feelings of helplessness and fear (Lepzcyk *et al.* 1990; Allen *et al.* 1992; Rakoczy 1997). Further thought may therefore be needed and larger-scale studies undertaken regarding the purpose and timing of pre-admission clinics. Reducing anxiety through regular manageable portions of information rather than providing it all at once, may prove more effective.

Any information should help the patient and family develop an understanding of the nature of impending surgery and foster the development of effective coping strategies. Individual coping styles must be considered and it is important to acknowledge that not all patients seek information but instead may demonstrate avoidance coping behaviours indicative of denial. This coping may be appropriate in the short term but could result in poor adjustment and possibly depression later. The challenge for the nurse is in identifying individual coping styles, adapting information accordingly and assisting in the development of more effective coping strategies. This task may be too complex to be undertaken in a group pre-admission clinic and may necessitate a more individualised approach.

In a small study of patients awaiting cardiac surgery half the sample said they would be interested to hear more about their illness and just over half would attend a support group if possible (Teo *et al.* 1998). Similar findings by Mark *et al.* (1997) concluded that a pre-surgical programme of support rather than a 'once only' visit may be beneficial. The importance of social support in the recovery process is well documented. Its impact is possibly through others encouraging positive health care practices (Hubbard *et al.* 1984; Moser 1994). A support group may offer an opportunity to communicate with others in a similar situation, enable comparisons and so help patients normalise their own experiences. Facilitation of the group by a health care professional offers additional support. Support groups for patients with chronic illness are well established but the concerns of relatives and caregivers must also be addressed.

Topics for patient education

Before pre-operative information can be given it is important to understand the type of information that may lead to positive outcome (Table 4.1). The period of time waiting for major surgery may be lengthy and the patient more concerned with the date of the operation than with details of the operation itself (Bengston *et al.* 1996). Similarly, patients on the waiting list for cardiac surgery often feel isolated and concerned that they may be forgotten (Davenport 1991). This uncertainty generates enormous anxiety and may exacerbate symptoms of decreased left ventricular function (Davenport 1991; Bengston *et al.* 1996). It is important to identify what the patient wants to know so that information is presented in a realistic and meaningful way and retention enhanced.

Table 4.1   Topics for patient education

A Relevant anatomy and physiology

B Procedural information
Description of the operation
Date of the operation
Description of the post-operative course – days in ITU, length of stay etc.
Reassurance that nurse present at all times
Means of communicating in ITU/preferred name
Activity levels after the operation
Breathing exercises or other exercises the patient will be asked to perform
Introduction of pain assessment tool
Eating and drinking
Description of catheters, IV lines and drains, IPPV, O_2 masks etc.
Medication and possible side-effects
Hospital visiting policy (less important)

C Sensory information
Discomfort associated with pain, nausea and thirst
Sensations associated with ITU environment, ventilatory assistance, suctioning etc.
Control of distressing sensations/discomfort – pain control, anti-emetics, moistening of mouth
Possible complications/associated risks and prolonged ITU stay
Possible meaning and explanation of symptoms experienced

D Post-operative issues and lifestyle changes
Return to social and employment activities, including sexual activity
Self-monitoring/self-management
(see Chapter 7 'Returning home')

If pre-operative education is to provide benefit to the patient and family, strategies should be used to enhance these benefits. Within the current philosophy of patient empowerment, active participation in goal setting and the implementation of care is appropriate. Interestingly, in one experimental study which measured the impact of active patient involvement, there was an increase in satisfaction in those actively involved in the education programme but no significant difference in post-operative complications and surgical outcome between the two groups (Wong & Wong 1985).

Sex differences

Although there has been a great deal written regarding the need for information among patients waiting or following surgery, few studies have addressed the differing needs of men and women. Although studies involving small samples have found no difference in the information needs of men and women (Galloway *et al.* 1993; Jickling & Graydon 1997), a more recent study of 700 patients awaiting coronary revascularisation indicated that women had greater fears surrounding surgery, anaesthesia and post-operative pain. Conversely, men were more fearful of the economic disruption or perceived sexual relationship changes (Koivula *et al.* 2001). Another study of women recovering from cardiac surgery revealed that women experience greater fatigue, have more negative emotions and are concerned over a lack of sensation in their breast region (Moore 1995). This sex difference in post-operative recovery should be reflected in the pre-operative information given to patients.

Strategies for patient education

Verbal information alone is often poorly retained and a variety of media is often more effective. Verbal information may be usefully supplemented with written leaflets or videos. The use of leaflets, however, is not without problems. Some information dates very quickly and information sponsored by commercial companies may emphasise bias and self-interest while hospital-produced information is both time-consuming and costly to prepare. Computer packages or videotapes may be of use, as can hospital websites for specific information, even providing a virtual tour of the hospital. This is particularly useful for patients who must travel to another hospital, e.g. a tertiary referral centre, which may be some distance from their home.

The main advantage of pre-admission clinics may be in the assessment of the patient by the surgeon and the provision of information by the nurse specialist.

It is unrealistic, with current health care delivery, to expect any nursing assessment to be performed by the nurse responsible for the patient's post-operative care. In small units this may be achievable, enabling the surgical nurse to build up a trusting relationship with both patient and family. However, there is no research to support this and it is the quality of the information giving and the documentation which is likely to be the key factor in contributing to improved communication and in allaying patient anxiety.

Fitness for surgery

In a study of patients awaiting cardiac surgery, Fitzsimons *et al.* (2000) demonstrated reduced physical functioning during the waiting period, and not surprisingly in almost 80% of the sample this had led to a significant deterioration in quality of life. Recovery is affected by health perceptions, and those with lower levels of perceived health are less likely to be relieved of their symptoms of angina or breathlessness following interventions (Fitzsimons *et al.* 2000; Lindsay *et al.* 2001). As patients become more sedentary prior to cardiothoracic surgery, their fitness for surgery may be compromised further. Maintaining physical activity should be a priority, yet as angina or breathlessness frequently increase during the wait for surgery, this will inevitably pose problems. Services for surgery must be maintained in order to reduce lengthy waiting periods and their significant detrimental impact on health outcome.

The long periods of waiting for surgery are likely to persist in the UK for some time and ways to use this time positively should be sought. The development of secondary prevention clinics should be considered, where secondary prevention advice including symptom management and smoking cessation could be given possibly influencing later surgical outcome. Results of a randomised controlled trial utilising a 'shared care' approach of monthly health education and motivational interviewing by a specialist nurse and practice nurse, resulted in a significant reduction in risk factors for CHD and operative risk and demonstrated an improvement in general health status (McHugh *et al.* 2001). Similar models have proved successful in chronic disease management such as asthma or diabetes. For patients awaiting cardiothoracic surgery, care is generally viewed as an issue for the acute secondary care sector. Yet the primary care setting is ideal for any pre-operative nursing intervention although there are developmental issues for those involved. Table 4.2 provides a useful guide for patient assessment.

Another strategy includes the use of a telephone support service to provide a more cost-effective and cost-efficient model of care. Telephone helplines have been widely used to provide up-to-date information, with individualised responses (Lindsay *et al.* 1995) and indeed this model is reflected in the NHS Direct service, providing reliable information to patients about their condition and treatment and advice regarding when to seek further medical help (DoH 1997).

The scarcity of resources reinforces the need for valid research and the piloting and evaluation of any proposed innovative model of care is crucial. Before any new care model is implemented cost should be considered together with the efficiency and effectiveness of the service delivered.

Physiological assessment

The waiting period for surgery should not just address patient education, but also allow time for nursing assessment, identification of any deficits and maximise the physical status. Optimising cardiorespiratory status to enhance recovery from surgery is particularly important. Each patient assessment should involve full coverage of the patient's physical and psychosocial status. Physical assessment will entail a review of all systems and will identify problems that may have particular significance for the current period of hospitalisation in terms of risk reduction. In reality the type of physical assessment carried out by nurses will be dictated by local practice and culture of the organisation. It is beyond the remit of

Table 4.2 Coronary heart disease: secondary prevention assessment

Target	Assessment tool	Progress
Smoking habit (smoking cessation)	Consumption	
Alcohol intake: females <1 unit/day males <2 units/day	Consumption	
Diet (5 portions fruit/vegetables/day)	3-day patient recall	
Blood cholesterol: HDL >1.0 mmol/l LDL <3.0 mmol/l	Fasting blood level	
Fasting blood glucose (<7.0 mmol/l)	Fasting blood level	
Blood pressure: <140/85 mmHg diabetics <130/80 mmHg	Sphygmomanometer	
Body mass index (<25.0)	Weight (kg)/Height (m^2)	
Waist girth: females <80 cm males <94 cm	Waist measurement	
Physical activity (regular aerobic activity of 30–40 min, 3–5 times/week)	Patient diary	
Functional ability	Exercise test/Duke activity status index. Symptoms: angina, breathlessness	
Improved quality of life	SF 36 questionnaire	
Psychosocial adjustment to chronic illness	PAIS questionnaire	
Stress management (no depression, functions well in all aspects of life)	HAD score	

this text to give a comprehensive account of how such an assessment should proceed. There are some excellent textbooks addressing this topic and suggestions are made at the end of this chapter.

Diagnostic tests are now widely available to provide an accurate assessment of the cardiac status (see Table 4.3). Although some of these tests will have been used to assist with the original diagnosis, they may also be useful to complete a physiological assessment and stratify post-operative risk. In patients undergoing

Table 4.3 Diagnostic tests for cardiac assessment

Diagnostic test	Description	Information gained	Nursing implications
Electrocardiogram	Recording of the conduction of the heart from various views	■ Characteristic patterns associated with ischaemia, injury, infarction and muscle mass size	■ No special preparation
Chest X-ray	Radiographic picture of the thorax	■ Cardiac shadow, left ventricular hypertrophy, cardiomegaly, pulmonary congestion/pleural effusion	■ No special preparation
Ambulatory (holter) monitoring	24 hour, 12 lead ECG recording. Monitor is worn with a strap around the body	■ Silent ischaemia or arrhythmias suggestive of ischaemia ■ Conduction abnormalities	■ Avoid showering, getting the box wet ■ Record diary throughout, noting symptoms of chest pain, palpitations, dizziness etc.
Exercise tolerance test (stress test, treadmill tests, exercise ECG)	Using a recognised protocol (usually the Bruce protocol) the patient walks on the treadmill and the slope and speed are increased at 2–3 minute intervals. Constant monitoring of ECG, HR and BP demonstrate the physiological response to exercise. The rate of perceived exertion is also recorded	■ Exercise-induced myocardial ischaemia demonstrated through ST segment changes ■ Limitation by HR or rate of perceived exertion (RPE) may relate more to deconditioning than to myocardial ischaemia	■ Patient must be aware that they can ask to stop the test ■ False positives may be found among women more frequently ■ Should not be used in presence of LBBB

Contd

Table 4.3 *Contd*

Diagnostic test	Description	Information gained	Nursing implications
Transthoracic echocardiography	High-frequency sound waves sent from a transducer echo off the heart structure to produce the picture of the heart	■ Useful to determine the cause of chest pain, valvular heart disease or cardiomyopathies (hypertrophic and dilated) ■ Estimates cardiac muscle mass, ejection fraction, end-diastolic and end-systolic volume ■ Ventricular wall motion, aneurysm, heart valve anatomy, blood flow, pressure gradients and pericardial effusions may also be detected	■ No special preparation ■ Patient will lie on an examination table usually tipped slightly onto their side ■ Patient may need to understand when to breathe in or out ■ Approx. 5 minutes for the test
Transoesophageal echocardiography	High-frequency sound waves are sent from a transducer that is attached to the distal end of a gastroscope and inserted into the oesophagus	■ Detailed size, shape and movement of the heart muscle ■ Dissection of the thoracic aorta ■ Heart valve dysfunction ■ Intracardiac thrombi ■ Cardiac/pericardial mass	■ Local anaesthetic to back of throat ■ Nothing orally for 4 hours prior to the test ■ IV cannula to administer mild relaxant ■ ECG monitor throughout ■ Small probe inserted into oesophagus ■ The test takes approx. 5 minutes
Coronary angiogram	Catheter inserted into coronary arteries, contrast medium injected	■ Used to establish a diagnosis of CHD in those with suspected angina ■ LV function and coronary arteries ■ Intracoronary pressures	■ Nothing orally 4 hours prior ■ Arterial puncture site – usually femoral or radial ■ Period of bed rest (approx. 4 hours) depending upon size of cannula and incision site

Right heart catheterisation	■ Catheter inserted into the right side of the heart	■ Intracardiac pressures of the right side of the heart ■ Cardiac output ■ Nothing orally 4 hours prior ■ Venous puncture site, usually femoral
Pulmonary arterial catheterisation	■ Insertion of a balloon-tipped catheter into the pulmonary artery	■ Left and right ventricular filling pressures ■ Cardiac output ■ Mixed venous oxygen sampling ■ Calculation of systemic and pulmonary vascular resistance ■ Haemodynamic status should be monitored carefully, e.g. in ICU
Nuclear imaging	■ Radioactive substance given. Myocardial perfusion is increased through pharmacological intervention (such as adenosine, dobutamine or dipyridamole) followed by thallium imaging	■ Presence and size of myocardial infarction or areas of poor perfusion. Normal uptake when resting, abnormal on exercise, indicates the blood flow is inadequate for exercising myocardium. Not normal at rest or on exercise, indicates part of the heart is permanently damaged and will not be resolved by revascularisation ■ Useful test for people who are unable to exercise, e.g. people with arthritis, CVA, PVD or with heart conduction problems such as LBBB ■ After exercise imaging, leave room for 3–4 hours (during which time caffeine should not be taken as it is an antagonist of adenosine) prior to repeat imaging ■ Adenosine should be avoided in asthmatics as it may induce bronchospasm
Carotid Doppler studies	■ Doppler recordings used to assess carotid flow	■ Useful in preparation for surgery ■ Risk of CVA in the post-operative period is increased with carotid artery atherosclerosis

Table 4.4   Examples of diagnostic tests prior to thoracic surgery

Diagnostic test	Description	Indications	Nursing implications
Bronchoscopy	Endoscopic view of the tracheobronchial tree using either flexible fibreoptic scope, rigid scope or laser bronchoscope	■ Diagnostic (sometimes biopsy) ■ May be therapeutic for haemoptysis, foreign bodies, stenosis. Laser used to reduce tumour size. More therapeutic bronchoscopic procedures hold promise for the future.	■ Nothing orally for 6 hours prior. Usually performed under local with sedation. Topical anaesthetic agent sprayed to throat ■ Observe haemodynamic and respiratory status during and following ■ Complications may include pneumothorax, bleeding, cardiac arrhythmias and worsening hypoxaemia ■ Introduce fluids gradually around 2 hours following procedure
Computerised axial tomography (CAT scan)	Non-invasive cross sectional anatomical view of soft tissues and bone which is more accurate than X-ray in detecting tumours	■ Diagnostic and staging of tumours. Able to detect hilar and mediastinal lymph nodes ■ High-resolution CT useful in bronchiectasis and interstitial lung disease	■ Jewellery and belts should be removed ■ No discomfort usually during procedure although position may increase breathlessness ■ Prepare patient for noise of the scanner

Magnetic resonance imaging (MRI)	■ Non-invasive, Patient placed in strong magnetic field. Microwave radio signal then beamed through body which interacts with hydrogen. These atoms then emit this absorbed energy to generate an image ■ An image can be constructed of the various densities of body tissues. Various views can be obtained, e.g. longitudinal and three-dimensional. Most useful where soft tissues involved. Provides good images of mediastinum and chest wall	■ No X-rays involved. Although magnetic field used this is harmless ■ Reassurance needed regarding noise ■ Patient may feel claustrophobic ■ All metal objects should be removed before procedure ■ Contraindicated where patients have implanted electronic devices
Positron emission tomography (PET) with fluorodeoxyglucose (FDG)	■ A positron-emitting isotope is tagged to a compound (usually glucose) and then injected. A PET scanner then measures not simply anatomical structures but metabolic/biochemical activity of the cells ■ Diagnostic. Useful to detect and stage malignant cells (these take up more of the compound, appearing brighter on images) and to evaluate effects of therapy ■ Scanning of whole body usually performed	■ Loose-fitting clothes worn; water only given ■ Radioactive drug administered intravenously or inhaled. Radioactive dose is very small and is quickly eliminated ■ Fluids encouraged following procedure to help with elimination
Mediastinoscopy	■ A rigid scope is used to allow inspection of mediastinum via small incision above suprasternal notch ■ Usually to determine mediastinal involvement in lung cancer when enlarged nodes seen on CT or MRI scans. A biopsy is taken	■ Observe for signs of possible haemorrhage and pneumothorax which may occur
Mediastinotomy	■ Direct exposure of lymph nodes through incision in second intercostal space on selected side ■ May involve opening of pleura to inspect hilum ■ Facilitates sampling of lymph nodes in the anterior mediastinum which are somewhat inaccessible with mediastinoscopy ■ Lymphatic spread to these nodes from left upper lobe tumour	■ Observe for signs of possible haemorrhage. A chest drain is inserted and connected to an underwater seal

Contd

Table 4.4 *Contd*

Diagnostic test	Description	Indications	Nursing implications
Transthoracic biopsy	Biopsy needle inserted in to the lungs and position confirmed by fluoroscopy or CT scan	■ Diagnostic for histology of tumours in lung periphery ■ Usually in patients not for surgery but performed to determine therapy. Possible false negatives	■ Pneumothorax and haemoptysis are possible complications ■ Chest X-ray usually performed following procedure to rule out pneumothorax
Open lung biopsy	Small specimen of lung tissue obtained through a small thoracotomy incision under general anaesthesia	■ For diagnostic purposes. One lung anaesthesia used ■ May be performed using a limited thoracotomy approach or using thoracoscopy (VATS approach)	■ Chest drain inserted ■ Principles of care as for any thoracotomy patient
Thoracoscopy	A rigid thoracoscope used which is inserted into the pleural space	■ May involve only a small stab incision with small volume of air introduced, separating pleura (local or general anaesthesia) ■ Intercostal access allows one or more resection biopsies to be taken ■ Video-assisted thoracoscopy may be preferred because of better visualisation (one lung anaesthesia needed)	■ Chest drain inserted ■ Principles of care as for any thoracotomy patient but shorter hospital stay usually compared with biopsy with limited thoracotomy

lung resection for malignancy, careful explanation may be needed regarding the many tests often requested for both diagnosis and staging of the tumour (see Table 4.4).

Cardiorespiratory assessment

Thorough assessment of the cardiorespiratory status of all patients should be undertaken prior to major surgery. While there have been advances in surgical techniques, patients are now often sicker and older. There may be more diffuse disease and co-morbidity is increasingly common presenting a real challenge for the surgical nurse.

A further important element of the pre-operative assessment is to determine which medications are being taken. Patients awaiting cardiothoracic surgery may have been taking aspirin and this should be stopped approximately one week prior to surgery to avoid post-operative bleeding. Warfarin should be stopped four days prior to surgery. When the risk of thrombotic disorders is very high, intravenous heparin or low molecular weight heparin is often given. This can be easily reversed for surgery yet prevents the risk of clot formation.

In patients with respiratory problems, glucocorticoid therapy may have been a part of the treatment regimen. The medical staff will need to determine the degree of adrenal suppression and ensure that the patient is capable of a normal adaptive stress response in order to avoid circulatory collapse post-operatively. Any provision of peri-operative glucocorticoids coverage must account for the patient's pre-operative glucocorticoid dose as well as the duration and severity of surgery or other stress (Lefor 1999), but for major surgery a dose of hydrocortisone from 100 to 150 mg per day for 2 to 3 days may be needed.

Cardiac assessment

Maximising the cardiac status can improve outcome from surgery and the elective pre-operative use of the intra-aortic balloon pump (IABP) pre-operatively may be effective for patients with poor left ventricular function or to control ischaemia in the elderly (Christenson *et al.* 1997). Used pre-operatively on high-risk patients with poor left ventricular function, myocardial ischaemia or a left main stem stenosis greater than 70%, the IABP can reduce operative time, improve cardiac output, reduce the time in intensive care and the overall hospital stay (Christenson *et al.* 1999). However, as IABP therapy is associated with its own complications it should be reserved for those patients who already have a high operative risk.

Cardiovascular disease is a leading cause of death and the fact that patients awaiting thoracic surgery may also have either diagnosed or undiagnosed coronary heart disease substantially increases their risk of a peri-operative myocardial infarction (MI) or cardiac death (Mangano & Goldman 1995). For those with diagnosed CHD, diagnostic tests (see Table 4.3) will be performed to assess cardiovascular function prior to any surgery and to stratify risk. However, patients may have undiagnosed CHD and so another important aspect of the physical assessment is to use good history taking to reveal symptoms indicative of angina, a previous MI, heart failure or cerebrovascular accident (CVA) when further diagnostic testing may be useful.

Any identified myocardial ischaemia in the person awaiting thoracic surgery, should be investigated further and it is usually sufficient to commence anti-anginal medication. However, in some instances, percutaneous transluminal angioplasty or coronary artery bypass grafting may be necessary before the patient is able to tolerate thoracic surgery.

Heart disease may occur secondary to a chronic lung disease. The strain placed upon the right side of the heart from pulmonary hypertension may lead to heart failure and the risk to the person undergoing thoracic surgery is increased. When heart failure is present in the person awaiting cardiac or thoracic surgery, this should be stabilised first and again medical treatment is usually sufficient.

Respiratory assessment

Maximising respiratory status is also important. The presence of a chronic lung disease in someone undergoing cardiac surgery is associated with post-operative pulmonary complications, a prolonged period of respiratory support, a longer intensive care unit stay and increased mortality (Cohen *et al.* 1995). Moreover, many patients with non-small-cell lung cancer will also have COPD increasing risk further.

In thoracic surgery many studies have been carried out to define levels of pre-operative lung function, which are physiologically compatible with lung resection. Pulmonary function tests are usually evaluated carefully in the pre-operative patient but there is controversy about their predictive value. There is increasing evidence to show that spirometry may not be as useful at predicting operative risk as once thought. Furthermore, where $PaCO_2$ is elevated in patients with pulmonary disease this is not seen as a risk factor in patients for lung resection (Kearney *et al.* 1994; Wisser *et al.* 1998). Gass and Olsen (1986) suggest that an increased risk of pulmonary complications is associated with a forced expiratory volume in one second (FEV_1) or forced vital capacity (FVC) of less than 70% of the predicted value, or a ratio of FEV_1 to FVC of less than 65%. Many surgeons agree with Goldstraw (1987) in that the predicted post-operative FEV_1 should exceed 800 ml. Patients with a post-operative FEV_1 greater than 40% of predicted rate are viewed as low risk for pneumonectomy. FEV_1 is usually related to total exhaled FVC. The ratio of FEV_1 to FVC may be reduced in the presence of airway obstruction but is normal in restrictive pulmonary disease. Although pulmonary function tests may not be routine in all cases, patients with a history of smoking or dyspnoea who are undergoing coronary bypass surgery and patients undergoing lung resection will have these done. More sophisticated tests may also be requested, including, for example, ventilation/perfusion scans and gas transfer tests.

Staging in patients with lung cancer

There are four major histological types, and identification is crucial as this will guide treatment. Small-cell tumours (20% of cases) develop mainly in the central airways, invade rapidly and are mostly associated with smoking, especially in women. By the time this tumour is diagnosed there is usually widespread dissemination and combination chemotherapy is the treatment of choice with surgery rarely an option.

Non-small-cell tumours include:

- Squamous: 40–70% of lung tumours, a slow-growing tumour developing centrally in the major bronchi
- Adenocarcinoma: 5–15% of lung tumours, developing in the lung periphery
- Large cell: 7–10% of lung tumours, developing in the lung apex or periphery

In patients with lung cancer an international staging system is available which assists medical staff in the decision-making process regarding therapeutic intervention (Mountain 1997). This TNM staging system considers three areas including tumour size (T), nodal involvement (N) and possible metastatic spread (M). A coding system is used for stage grouping, and tumours in the early stages would be coded as follows:

- **Stage IA (T1 N0 M0):** where the tumour is less than 3 cm involving the lung or visceral pleura with no nodal involvement or metastatic spread.
- **Stage IB (T2 N0 M0):** where tumour is greater than 3 cm which may involve the main bronchus more than 2 cm distal to the carina and/or visceral pleura. Although there may be associated pressure/obstructive problems there is no nodal involvement or metastatic spread.
- **Stage IIA (T1 N1 M0):** where the tumour is smaller than 3 cm with involvement of hilar nodes on the same side but no distant metastatic spread.
- **Stage IIB (T2 N1 M0):** where the tumour is greater than 3 cm possibly involving the main bronchus (>2 cm distal to the carina), visceral pleura and/or with associated pressure/obstructive problems but no distant metastatic spread. This stage would also include a tumour of any size directly invading the chest wall, diaphragm, mediastinal pleura, parietal pericardium and main bronchus (<2 cm distal to but not involving the carina) but with no nodal involvement or metastatic spread (T3 N0 M0).

If histology identifies a non-small-cell carcinoma as above then surgical resection is a real possibility. Tumours at stages III and IV, where there is much more nodal involvement with or without distant metastatic spread, are usually too advanced for surgery and the prognosis is poor.

The above staging system is appropriate only for non-small-cell tumours. Small-cell (oat cell) tumours are classified as either limited, if confined to one hemithorax with or without contralateral hilar or ipsilateral supraclavicular lymph node involvement, or extensive, where the disease has spread further.

Patients presenting for surgery with lung cancer may be very healthy and vigorous, or may have significant medical complexities including severe metabolic disturbances and advanced organ impairment due to their malignancy or its treatment (Schmiesing & Fischer 2001). Weakness may be profound in some patients and some problems may have been precipitated by chemotherapy and radiation regimens pre-operatively. Radiation, for example, may cause pulmonary fibrosis, pneumonitis and pleural effusions and it may be necessary to perform arterial blood gas analysis, spirometry, ventilation perfusion scans and diffusing capacity. Failure to detect pulmonary problems as a result of cancer treatment may result in serious pulmonary compromise post-operatively.

Some patients are accepted for surgery with no formal measurement of pulmonary function and this may be acceptable for patients with a local lesion and no history of past or present pulmonary disease. However, even when spirometry results are less than ideal, the risk from surgery may be acceptable in some cases. Although existing pulmonary disease increases risk, in one retrospective study 107 patients tolerated non-cardiac surgery relatively well despite severe COPD on spirometry (Kroenke *et al.* 1992). The challenge for the future is illustrated by the sobering fact that of 100 patients with lung cancer, only 8 will be alive five years after presentation and only 4 after ten years (Ghosh & Latimer 1999).

As spirometry may not be performed on all patients the nurse's observations during assessment are important in identifying clinical variables, e.g. dyspnoea, which may contribute towards predicting post-operative cardiopulmonary complications. This may also avoid the need for spirometry.

Pulmonary risk and smoking
A recent history of smoking may result in problems with mucociliary functioning post-operatively with possible retention of secretions in both cardiac and thoracic patients. It appears that if smoking cessation before surgery is to be beneficial then this must be at least eight weeks before surgery. In a study of 200 smokers for coronary bypass surgery there was a lower risk of pulmonary complications in those who had stopped at least eight weeks prior to surgery than among current smokers (Warner *et al.* 1996), with patients who quit less than eight weeks before surgery having a higher risk than current smokers.

Many patients may be long-term smokers and pack-years should be calculated. Although there may have been periods when there was abstinence, each period of smoking needs to be calculated and then added for total pack-years. The number of pack-years gives some indication regarding risk for development of chronic obstructive pulmonary disease. It is calculated as follows:

$$\frac{\text{Number smoked each day}}{20} \times \text{Years of smoking} = \text{Pack-years}$$
$$(> 15 = \text{significant risk})$$

Pulmonary risk and obesity
There is no obvious pulmonary risk associated with obesity although risk for thrombo-embolism following surgery is increased. Obese patients often have difficulty with ventilation in the immediate post-operative period but the incidence of pneumonia and atelectasis is similar to that for non-obese patients following thoracic surgery. Even the presence of obstructive sleep apnoea (OSA) does not necessarily preclude surgery so long as nasal continuous positive airway pressure is utilised before and following surgery (Rennotte *et al.* 1995). It is worth noting that OSA may not have been diagnosed and it is suggested that unexpected post-operative deaths occurring at night may be due to OSA (Rosenberg & Kehlet 1991).

Patients with a history of chronic lung disease must be assessed and their pulmonary function improved as much as possible. Although patients may not have been previously diagnosed with asthma/COPD, some may show some airway reversibility following administration of a β_2 agonist. The nurse must therefore obtain details regarding history of cough, sputum production and possible dyspnoea on exertion. Where symptoms are present a combination of bronchodilators, physiotherapy, antibiotics, smoking cessation and corticosteroids have been shown to reduce the risk of post-operative complications. Although patients may have a history of bronchial asthma this does not necessarily increase the risk of pulmonary complications (Warner *et al.* 1996) so long as the peak expiratory flow rate is greater than 80% of the predicted or patient's personal best. If the peak flow is less than optimum a short rescue course of corticosteroids may be prescribed. Spirometry and peak expiratory flow rates can be easily obtained by the nurse.

Lung function in obstructive pulmonary disease

Spirometry   A spirometer is used to help diagnose and monitor asthma and COPD and to monitor progress. Simple electronic devices are available which are easy to use. Following a maximum inspiratory effort the patient makes a sustained maximum expiratory effort through the mouthpiece of the spirometer which is maintained until no more air can be removed. Spirometry is able to measure the following:

■ **Forced vital capacity (FVC):** the maximum volume of air inhaled and exhaled from the lungs made up of inspiratory reserve volume, tidal volume and expiratory reserve volume
■ **Forced expiratory volume in 1 second (FEV$_1$):** the proportion of the FVC removed in the first second

From the above two measurements the FEV$_1$-to-FVC ratio can be calculated. This is a more useful measurement than the FEV$_1$ or FVC alone. The ratio is a much better measure of airflow limitation and is related to height, age and sex of the patient. Where airflow is good the ratio should be at least 70%. As an example, let FEV$_1$ = 3.0 litres and FVC = 3.8 litres. Then:

$$\frac{FEV_1}{FVC} = 79\%$$

In obstructive disorders,

■ High intrathoracic pressures generated by forced expiration cause premature closure of the airways with trapping of air in the chest
■ FEV$_1$ is reduced much more than FVC
■ FEV$_1$/FVC ratio is reduced

Peak expiratory flow rate (PEFR)   Peak expiratory flow rate is the greatest flow that can be sustained for 10 milliseconds on forced expiration starting from maximum inspiration. It is a simple, quantitative and reproducible measure to perform, most often used in asthma for monitoring progress. A Wright Peak Flow Meter or Mini-Wright Meter is used for this test and the measurement is in litres per minute. Normal PEFR is around 400–650 l/min in healthy adults although this should be compared to the predicted value or patient's best. Prior to surgery, PEFR should be greater then 80% of the predicted or patient's personal best. The best of three measurements is recorded, calculated as follows:

$$\frac{\text{Current PEFR}}{\text{Best}} \times 100$$

For example:

$$\frac{550}{650} \times 100 = 85\%$$

PEFR rate is reduced in:

- Asthma and COPD
- Upper airway tumours

A reduced FVC without airflow obstruction may be evidence of disease of the thoracic cage or lung parenchyma (i.e. restrictive lung diseases where there is reduced compliance but little or no obstruction).

Any abnormalities detected with either spirometry or peak expiratory flow rate values should be reported to the medical staff for investigation including possible reversibility testing.

Nutritional assessment

The patient awaiting cardiothoracic surgery may be cachectic and malnourished because of longstanding heart failure, cancer or chronic respiratory failure and consequently has a substantially increased risk of complications following surgery (Paccagnella *et al.* 1994). Additionally, difficulty in swallowing, reduced appetite, vomiting or diarrhoea are symptoms frequently associated with chronic lung or heart disease and side-effects of treatment for malignancy. Poor nutrition will lead to respiratory muscle atrophy and poor reserves for the increased work of breathing, difficulty weaning from intermittent positive pressure ventilation, delayed wound healing, infection and poor functional ability, and is therefore likely to compound the post-operative period. Patients with chronic lung disease or severe heart failure may have right-sided heart failure leading to abnormal liver function, as well as poor nutritional status, whereas patients on longstanding diuretic therapy may have low potassium levels. The pre-operative assessment should note any abnormalities such as abnormal electrolytes, low albumin levels or raised prothrombin times and correct these prior to surgery.

The nursing assessment invariably includes questions regarding nutrition and alcohol consumption and detailed information needs to be obtained in this area (Table 4.5). Prior to cardiothoracic surgery the nurse needs to obtain specific data about dietary intake, including quantity and quality of daily meals. This is an ideal health promotion opportunity where the nurse can identify knowledge deficits which can be addressed later. Weight loss and hypoalbuminaemia are predictors of poor surgical outcome. Poor dietary intake may increase risk considerably because of resulting poor immune function, and benefit may be gained from a pre-operative inpatient stay in order to optimise nutritional status which may include both enteral and parenteral nutrition (Paccagnella *et al.* 1994). As far as surgery and wound complications are concerned, it is recent dietary intake that is most important (Haydock & Hill 1987). It is possible that pre-operative nutritional support may be required for at least seven days in the undernourished patient.

Table 4.5   Factors to consider in nutritional assessment

- Body weight $<20\,km/m^2$ or $>30\,kg/m^2$
- Involuntary loss or gain of weight of more than:
  10% of usual body weight within past six months, or
  5% of usual body weight within one month
- A weight of 20% over or under ideal body weight
- Chronic lung disease
- Chronic heart failure
- Alteration to usual dietary intake, possibly due to increasing breathlessness, anxiety
- Alteration in medication
- Usual fruit and vegetable intake
- Nutritional supplements
- Blood sampling for albumin, clotting times

Ideal body weight, serum albumin and arm muscle circumference have all been used to evaluate nutritional status although it has been suggested that the latter two may be unreliable markers. A body mass index (BMI) $<18\,kg/m^2$ may indicate malnourishment and the need for further nutritional assessment. Weight loss is a correlate of protein energy malnutrition (PEM) and a loss $>10\%$ indicates significant PEM (Hill 1992). Weight lost compared with the patient's usual body weight may therefore better identify those who may be compromised, with a 10% loss from usual body weight requiring further investigation (McClave & Snider 1999). Caution needs to be exercised in the presence of oedema as weight values will be unreliable and may hide an underlying nutritional deficit.

Conversely, obesity (BMI $>30\,kg/m^2$) also influences the post-operative recovery period, increasing the risk of mediastinitis (Zacharias & Habib 1996; Jakob *et al.* 2000), leg wound infection (Thomas *et al.* 1995; Englemann *et al.* 1999) and pulmonary problems. A weight-reducing diet may be required under the supervision of a dietitian to ensure that all nutritional needs are met.

Special pre-operative issues

Age

A significant number of patients presenting for cardiac and thoracic surgery will be elderly, and maximising surgical outcome may require specific attention. Changes to the heart occur with age. Not only is there an increased incidence of hypertension and coronary heart disease but there are also changes to the myocardium itself. Increased stiffness of the great arteries increases afterload and changes in excitation–contraction coupling lead to prolonged contraction and myocardial stiffness. Diastolic dysfunction results, cardiac output falls and myocardial oxygen consumption increases (McConachie 2002). The myocardium is more sensitive to ischaemia in the older person and the use of strategies to improve myocardial preservation and possibly the pre-operative use of the intra-aortic balloon pump (IABP) should be considered.

Arrhythmias are not uncommon with advancing age, with atrial fibrillation affecting approximately 4% of people over 60. This figure is higher still when combined with lung or heart disease, heart failure or diabetes. Age is also associated with the development of collagenous tissue in the heart's conduction pathways resulting in sinus and atrioventricular node disorders with sinus bradycardia, sick sinus syndrome and heart blocks arising.

Alterations to the respiratory system also occur with age. The lungs become less compliant, thereby increasing the work of breathing. Respiratory muscle strength diminishes, although this appears strongly correlated to nutritional status and the cardiac index. Despite these changes, the respiratory system is capable of maintaining an adequate gaseous exchange. In the presence of an acute illness, however, the respiratory system reserve declines and there appears to be a decrease in the sensitivity of the respiratory centre to hypoxia and hypercapnia (Janssens *et al.* 1999). The elderly are able to increase their respiratory rate but are not able to alter their tidal volume in response. Another important factor when caring for the elderly person undergoing cardiothoracic surgery includes their blunted laryngeal reflexes and therefore the increased likelihood of aspiration during anaesthesia (McConachie 2002).

Age-related changes to other major body systems that can impact upon the pre-operative course also occur. For example, there is a fall in the glomerular filtration rate of the kidneys, the renal tubular function declines and there is a slight reduction in hepatic function. These issues result in what is frequently observed as a slower post-operative recovery and therefore should be anticipated from the pre-operative assessment. Adequate preparation can then be given to explain these issues.

Anaemia

Addressing nutritional needs that may influence clotting will enhance post-operative recovery and possibly also reduce the need for blood transfusions. The need for transfusion following surgery depends largely upon two main variables. One is blood volume lost during the surgical procedure itself whereas the other relates to individual ability to withstand blood loss and this can be influenced by pre-operative preparation. A patient with a low packed cell volume at the time of surgery is more likely to bleed. Pre-operative anaemia can be easily detected and is more common in the elderly, those with poor nutritional status, in malignant disease, where approximately 50% of patients may be anaemic (Mercurialli & Inghilleri 1998), and in other chronic illness such as lung disease. Correction of anaemia and promotion of erythropoiesis may be achieved in the pre-operative wait for surgery. Encouraging a healthy diet, prescribing oral iron supplements or even the intravenous administration of iron may be effective.

Erythropoietin, a growth factor for red blood cells, is normally specifically secreted in response to tissue hypoxia. Intravenous recombinant human erythropoietin (rHuEPO) a pharmacological agent, stimulates erythropoiesis and has been shown to be a useful adjunct to iron therapy to treat pre-operative anemia. It has also been successfully used to enable autologous blood transfusion (Helm *et al.* 1993; Mercurialli & Inghilleri 1998), of particular value in reducing the financial cost of using donor blood while preserving scarce resources. The period of time required for successful treatment may be as little as two weeks. However, this form of treatment in itself is costly, and better use of it may be through pre-operative risk stratification to determine those most likely to require post-operative blood transfusion.

Issues regarding risk and outcome

The risk that patients are exposed to when undergoing cardiac and thoracic surgery is difficult to predict accurately. Measurement of risk is an inexact science and although risk assessment tools are available these can only offer a guide regarding patient suitability for surgery. The risk of an untoward event occurring before, during or following surgery will depend on a host of different factors. Many of these are unrelated to the patient. There is an expectation, for instance, that all medical and nursing personnel will have the appropriate expertise to care for patients effectively, and that all support staff will be diligent in their duties in ensuring that the hospital environment is safe. Health care in the twenty-first century is not risk-free, however, and more individuals are aware of the fallibility of the health care system (Dalziel 2001). Most organisations are working towards ensuring that an effective clinical risk management policy is in place so that risk is reduced as far as possible.

Most procedures in cardiothoracic surgery are major and invasive in nature and traumatise the body significantly, not least in terms of haemodynamic and pulmonary instability. Moreover, patients bring risk with them and it is important to be able to assess the degree of risk in this area so that decisions can be made about the most appropriate course of action. The final decision may be not to operate, or where surgery is still considered worthwhile, taking all appropriate steps to minimise risk further.

A number of risk assessment tools have been developed, and these are useful not only in giving patients and families insight into risk of complications and mortality, so important for gaining informed consent, but also for increasing the awareness of the health care team to high-risk patients for whom more aggressive therapy in the pre-, intra- or post-operative period may be beneficial (Bojar 1999). In health care systems under pressure, risk stratification will become increasingly important in the efficient use of health care resources. The risk to the patient of undergoing major surgery is well documented (Devereaux *et al.* 1999), although the means of determining risk to a specific patient is less well delineated and various tools have been developed to assist in identification of this risk. As most deaths are from cardiac disorders (Jones & deCossart 1999), some tools specifically predict the risk of a cardiac complication.

It is important, however, to recall how the pattern of surgery is changing. With advances in minimally invasive techniques the patient undergoing more conventional surgery is tending to be older with more complex disease. Age, while an important consideration, is no longer a contra-indication for surgery. Most risk stratification tools available are based on information in three important areas:

- Identification of factors independent of the disease, e.g. age, sex
- Presence of coexisting disease, i.e. co-morbidities
- Nature and extent of cardiac disease and urgency of surgery

Assessment tools

The following sections give an overview of some of the popular risk assessment tools. One problem in identifying the degree of risk with any certainty is that often there are multiple factors present and these may interact in complex ways to finally impact on outcome.

Goldman Multifactorial Cardiac Risk Index

The Goldman Multifactorial Cardiac Risk Index (Goldman *et al.* 1977; Goldman 1995) was designed to quantify the cardiovascular risk following non-cardiac surgery. A number of risk factors are identified and weighted to enable scoring (see Table 4.6). Although a high score is associated with high risk, because of the index's low sensitivity not all high-risk patients may be identified. Nevertheless, it is often used in thoracic surgery as morbidity and mortality from cardiovascular diseases are major complications of thoracic surgery.

Although there have been further attempts to assess cardiopulmonary risk following thoracic surgery (Epstein *et al.* 1993) through modification of the Goldman criteria index, these have not produced a reliable predictive tool that can be applied to diverse populations in different institutions (Melendez *et al.* 1998).

Parsonnet score

The Parsonnet score (Parsonnet *et al.* 1989) is applied to individuals with coronary heart disease and has been widely used in risk stratification for coronary artery bypass grafting (CABG) (Riley 1995; Lawrence *et al.* 2000). Objective and easily

Table 4.6(a)   Goldman risk scoring

Risk factor	Points
Raised JVP	11
Previous MI <6 months	10
Ventricular ectopics (>5/min)	7
Rhythm other than sinus or sinus + atrial premature beats on last pre-op. ECG	7
Age >70 years	5
Emergency operation	3
Severe aortic stenosis	3
Poor general condition, e.g. poor PaO_2, $PaCO_2$, creatinine	3
Intraperitoneal/intrathoracic operation or aortic surgery	3

Source: Goldman *et al.* 1977

Table 4.6(b)   Performance of risk index in practice

Points	Life threatening complications (%)	Cardiac deaths (%)
0–5	0.7	0.2
6–12	5	2
13–25	11	2
26+	20	56

Source: Goldman *et al.* 1977; Goldman 1995

obtainable data is used to stratify patients according to risk. This data includes, for example, age, sex, presence of co-morbidities such as diabetes or hypertension, chronic renal failure requiring dialysis, and left ventricular function (Table 4.7). This data is then weighted to produce a score.

Although, it has been suggested that the Parsonnet score may not be sufficiently reliable on its own for the assessment of risk (Pons *et al.* 1998), it has been useful in planning care, where patients with a high Parsonnet score (>20) were more likely to have an increased stay in the intensive care unit (Doering *et al.* 2001). Considering this, it would appear that the pre-operative status of the patient is more important for post-operative recovery than events such as the development of post-operative arrhythmias or haemodynamic instability. The Parsonnet scoring system could then be useful to tailor individual pre-operative information relating to length of time in hospital or the intensive care unit.

APACHE

Scores of severity of illness based on physiological response have also been developed and include an assessment of the severity of acute physiological disturbance (acute physiology and chronic health evaluation, APACHE) (Knaus *et al.* 1985). This index was developed from a database of 5815 intensive care admissions in the USA. It is more appropriate for the post-operative period in the

Table 4.7 Some components of the Parsonnet scoring model

Factor	Assigned weight
Male	1
Obesity >1.5 ideal body weight	3
Hypertension >140 mmHg systolic	3
Diabetes	3
Ejection fraction: good	0
fair	2
poor	4
Age: 70–74	7
75–79	12
>80 years	20
Redo operation	10
Valve surgery:	
Mitral	5
PAP >60 mmHg	8
Aortic	5
Pressure gradient >120 mmHg	7
CABG at time of valve surgery	2

intensive care unit (ICU) and can quantify the severity of illness and predict overall mortality for a group of patients. It cannot predict accurately the outcome in individual patients but allows useful comparisons between centres. It requires extensive collection of data, which limits its user friendliness.

APACHE II is a simplified measure of the original tool using 12 physiological measures combined with a measure of chronic health status but scoring requires extremely accurate information and this is often difficult to achieve.

TISS

A measure of therapeutic effect expended on a patient (therapeutic intervention scoring system, TISS) (Keene & Cullen 1983) grades the severity of illness through the use of therapeutic interventions to provide an evaluation of severity of illness in the ICU. For example, the score will be higher for someone requiring intermittent positive pressure ventilation (IPPV) and inotropic support over someone on continuous positive airway pressure (CPAP). This tool refers more to the post-operative period and is useful to predict days needed in ICU rather than patient outcome. APACHE, TISS and other similar tools are not designed to predict patient outcome but are used as scoring systems for administrative purposes regarding ICU beds.

Attempts have also been made to develop tools to predict risk relating to specific complications arising post-operatively in areas such as wound infection, pulmonary difficulties and nutritional deficit. These will be addressed in the relevant sections elsewhere.

Baseline assessment tools

Evaluation of functional status may also provide useful information as severe limitation of activity, such as being immobile in the pre-operative phase predicts post-operative risk of a cardiac event (Browner *et al.* 1992). Many patients will have experienced a range of symptoms including dyspnoea, pain and fatigue, with varying degrees of disability. Evaluation of functional status may not only contribute to risk assessment but also enable comparisons to be made when monitoring progress on follow-up visits. The New York Heart Association (NYHA) functional classification scale (Criteria Committee of the New York Heart Association 1979) is a relatively simple tool which assesses cardiovascular disability of patients (see Table 4.8(a)). The modified Borg scale (Burdon *et al.* 1982) provides information about the patient's perceived dyspnoea and may provide a useful baseline from which the nurse can make an objective assessment of future progress in patients with pulmonary problems (see Table 4.8(b)). The Medical Research Council (MRC) dyspnoea scale (Fletcher 1960) is used to monitor

Table 4.8(a) New York Heart Association functional classification scale

Class	Functionality
I	Patients with heart disease who have no symptoms of any sort. No limitation of physical activity. Ordinary physical activity does not cause undue fatigue, palpitation or dyspnoea
II	Slight limitation of physical activity. Comfortable at rest, but ordinary physical activity results in fatigue, palpitation or dyspnoea
III	Marked limitation of physical activity. Comfortable at rest, but less than ordinary activity causes fatigue, palpitation or dyspnoea
IV	Symptoms at rest. Unable to carry out any physical activity without discomfort

Table 4.8(b) Modified Borg scale (of perceived breathlessness)

Scale	Severity
0	None at all
0.5	Very, very slight (just noticeable)
1	Very slight
2	Slight
3	Moderate
4	Somewhat severe
5	Severe
6	
7	Very severe
8	
9	Very, very severe (almost maximum)
10	Maximum

Table 4.8(c)   Medical Research Council dyspnoea scale

Grade	Degree of breathlessness related to activities
0	Not troubled by breathlessness except on strenuous exercise
1	Short of breath when hurrying or walking up a slight hill
2	Walks slower than contemporaries on the level because of breathlessness, or has to stop for breath when walking at own pace
3	Stops for breath after walking about 100 m or after a few minutes on the level
4	Too breathless to leave the house, or breathless when dressing or undressing
5	Breathless at rest

patients with COPD (Bestall *et al.* 1999), and while linked to functional ability may not be sensitive enough to detect small changes in other pulmonary disorders (see Table 4.8(c)).

Psychosocial assessment

The cognitive decline which occurs in some patients, particularly the elderly, after cardiac surgery, is well documented (Hammon *et al.* 1997; Selnes *et al.* 1999), and despite improvements in surgical techniques the incidence has changed little over the past 15 years (Newman *et al.* 2001). Given that cognitions are a powerful determinant of behaviour and emotion, psychological factors may contribute to morbidity and mortality post-operatively. Indeed, psychosocial factors are known to be significant predictors of morbidity and mortality in cardiac patients (Moser & Dracup 1995; Lim *et al.* 1998), with social support as a coping resource enhancing physical and psychological well-being following cardiac surgery (Jenkins *et al.* 1994; Thoits 1995). There is a range of tools available – some disease-specific, others generic – which measure many of the variables associated with chronic illness. Although used extensively in research studies, many of these are too long and time consuming in their completion to be of use in clinical practice.

Given that a significant proportion of medical patients have been found to have psychological difficulties, including anxiety and depression (Royal College of Physicians and Royal College of Psychiatrists 1995), it is highly likely that so too will some patients presenting for surgery. Although many patients will view the prospect of cardiac surgery with some optimism it should not be assumed that psychosocial and emotional resources are strong enough to support coping through the recovery process. While there is an increasing volume of literature regarding the recovery of patients following cardiac surgery there is a dearth of literature regarding the experience of different groups following thoracic surgery. Anxiety and depression may be particularly troublesome in patients with chronic pulmonary disease and in patients undergoing surgery for malignancy.

Most risk-stratification tools outlined earlier do not include a psychosocial dimension, which, given the accumulating evidence regarding the role of psychosocial factors in recovery from surgery, makes it imperative that further research is conducted and tools developed to identify those at risk. Patients who show high scores for poor psychosocial adjustment and coping may benefit greatly from additional support perhaps including some form of psycho-therapeutic intervention pre- and post-operatively. Various intervention strategies have been successfully utilised, but again, while there is increasing evidence to support their use following cardiac surgery these need to be evaluated in patients following thoracic surgery.

Recognition of the importance of psychosocial variables is reflected in the volume of literature in this area. Cohen & Rodriguez (1995) offer a useful theoretical framework explaining how biological, cognitive, behavioural and social pathways may contribute to psychological difficulty in those with a physical disorder. This model is bi-directional in that any psychological disturbance resulting via these pathways may, through these same pathways, result in further pathology. There have been numerous attempts by nursing academics to devise appropriate theoretical frameworks to explain coping and many of these draw heavily on the transactional model of stress by Lazarus & Folkman (1984). These have been useful in guiding research and in assisting nurses to carry out psychosocial assessments and identify areas where psychosocial intervention may be required.

An appropriate framework can be useful in the cardiothoracic surgical setting enabling the nurse to predict those patients who require more intensive intervention both before and following surgery. Figure 4.1 offers a practical framework for such a psychosocial assessment incorporating the ideas of Cohen & Rodriguez and Lazarus & Folkman. Four key areas to be explored are identified. It is under the behavioural responses heading that coping is addressed, recognising that the patient's responses may reflect either problem-focused or emotional-focused coping. Inappropriate coping may be the result of difficulties in other areas, and strengthening psychosocial resources and teaching more effective ways of coping may contribute to improved outcome.

Using the HADS scale to identify those patients who require a more comprehensive assessment may also help. This is a 14-item scale that provides a simple, brief 'state' measure of both anxiety (seven items) and depression (seven items) (Zigmund & Snaith 1983), and in 100 medical outpatients, scores from 8 to 10 on each scale have been taken to indicate possible clinical disorder, and from 11 to 21 to indicate probable clinical disorder.

Evaluation of surgical success should be concerned not only with the short period following surgery but also with long-term follow-up, during which time the help of a skilled health worker may be needed. A framework can also be used to identify the level of information required by different types of individuals, to predict those individuals who may experience more pain after surgery, to develop more effective coping strategies for pain management (Shaw 1999), and in adjustment generally post-operatively. Before such claims can be made, however, more work is needed on the development and validation of an effective psychosocial assessment tool that could be used by nurses in the surgical setting.

The nurse has an important role to play in carrying out an effective pre-

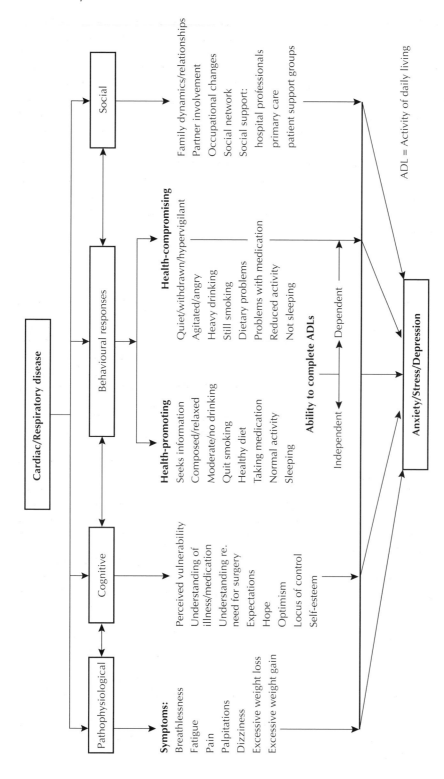

Fig. 4.1 Framework for psychosocial assessment.

operative assessment in patients undergoing cardiothoracic surgery. No patient is entirely free of risk as far as post-operative complications are concerned. Many cardiac and thoracic procedures are viewed by health staff as routine and often the post-operative course is uneventful. Patient discharge is earlier than ever before and the nurse is presented with the real challenge of preparing the patient both psychologically and physically in a much shorter period of time pre-operatively. But there is much that can go wrong and the experienced nurse must be aware of each possible eventuality together with the measures to be taken should these occur.

A comprehensive assessment will enable the nurse to identify factors which may contribute to the development of problems during the period of hospitalisation particularly following surgery and beyond discharge. An awareness of factors predicting post-operative risk will enable the health care team to target specific areas and to optimise the patient's general health.

References

Allen, M., Knight, C., Falk, C., Strung, V. (1992) Effectiveness of a preoperative teaching programme for cataract patients. *Journal of Advanced Nursing* **17**: 303–9.

Bengston, A., Herlitz, J., Karlsson, T. & Hjalmarson, A. (1996) Distress correlates with the degree of chest pain: a description of patients awaiting revascularisation. *Heart* **75**: 257–60.

Bergmann, P., Huber, S., Machler, H., Liebl, E. *et al.* (2000) Perioperative course of stress in patients confronting surgery. *The Internet Journal of Thoracic and Cardiovascular Surgery* **3**(2). Available at http://www.ispub.com/journals/ijtcvs.htm. Accessed 1 November 2002.

Bestall, J.C., Paul, E.A., Garrod, R., Garnham, R., Jones, P.W. & Wedzicha, J.A. (1999) Usefulness of the Medical Research Council (MRC) dyspnoea scale as a measure of disability in patients with chronic obstructive pulmonary disease. *Thorax* **54**(7): 581–6.

Billing, J., Arifi, A., Sharples, L., Tsui, S. & Nashef, S. (1996) Heart surgery management in UK patients: planned or crisis management? *Lancet* **347**(9000): 540–41.

Bojar, R.M. (1999) *Manual of Perioperative Care in Cardiac Surgery.* Blackwell Science, London.

Boore, J. (1978) *Information: A Prescription for Recovery.* Royal College of Nursing, London.

Browner, W.S., Li, J. & Mangano, D. (1992) In-hospital and long term mortality in male veterans following noncardiac surgery. The study of perioperative Ischaemia Research group. *Journal of the American Medical Association* **268**: 228–32.

Burdon, G.W., Juniper, E.F., Killian, K.J., Hargarve, F.E. & Campbell, E.J.M. (1982) The perception of breathlessness in asthma. *American Review of Respiratory Disease* **140**: 1021–7.

Christenson, J., Simonet, F., Badel, M. & Schuziger, M. (1997) Evaluation of preoperative intra-aortic balloon support in high risk coronary patients. *European Journal of Cardiothoracic Surgery* **11**: 1097–103.

Christenson, J., Simonet, F., Badel, P., Schuziger, M. (1999) Optimal timing of preoperative intra-aortic balloon pump support in high-risk coronary patients. *Annals of Thoracic Surgery* **68**: 934–99.

Chrousos, G.P. & Gold, P.W. (1992) The concepts of stress and stress system disorders: overview of physical and behavioural homeostasis. *Journal of the American Medical Association* **267**: 1244–52.

Cohen, A., Katz, M., Katz, R., Hauptman, E. & Schachner, A. (1995) Chronic obstructive pulmonary disease in patients undergoing coronary artery bypass grafting. *Journal of Thoracic and Cardiovascular Surgery* **109**: 574–81.

Cohen, S. & Rodriguez, M.S. (1995) Pathways linking affective disturbances and physical disorders. *Health Psychology* **14**(5): 374–80.

Colacchio, T.A., Yeager, M.P. & Hilderbrandt, L.W. (1994) Perioperative immuno-modulation in cancer surgery. *American Journal of Surgery* **167**(1): 174–9.

Craig, S.R., Leaver, H.A., Yap, P.L. *et al.* (2001) Acute phase response following minimal access and conventional thoracic surgery. *European Journal of Cardiothoracic Surgery* **20**: 455–63.

Criteria Committee of the New York Heart Association Inc. (1979) *Nomenclature and Criteria for the Diagnosis of the Heart and Great Vessels*, 8th edn. Little, Brown & Co., Boston.

Cupples, S. (1991) Effects of timing and reinforcement of preoperative education on knowledge and recovery of patients having coronary artery bypass graft surgery. *Heart and Lung* **20**(6): 654–60.

Dalziel, M. (2001) Governance as a local mechanism for the early detection and mini-mization of medical error: defining the role and methods of critical incident reporting, risk management and whistle blowing. In: Miles, A., Hill, A.P. & Hurwitz, B. (eds) *Clinical Governance and the NHS Reforms: Enabling Excellence or Imposing Control*. Aescu-lapius Medical Press, London.

Davenport, Y. (1991) The waiting period prior to cardiac surgery – when complicated by sudden cancellation. *Intensive Care Nurse* **7**: 105–13.

Devereaux, P., Ghali, W., Gibson, N. *et al.* (1999) Physician estimates of perioperative car-diac risk in patients undergoing noncardiac surgery. *Archives of Internal Medicine* **159**(7): 713–17.

Dhabhar, F.S., Miller, A.H., Stein, M., McEwen, B.S. & Spencer, R.L. (1994) Diurnal and acute stress-induced changes in distribution of peripheral leucocyte subpopulations. *Brain Behaviour and Immunity* **8**: 66–79.

Doering, L., Esmailian, F., Imperial-Perez, F. & Monsein, S. (2001) Determinants of intensive care unit length of stay after coronary artery bypass graft surgery. *Heart and Lung* **30**(1): 9–17.

DoH (Department of Health) (1997) *The New NHS: Modern, Dependable*. HMSO, London.

Doogue, M., Brett, C. & Elliott, J. (1997) Life and death on the waiting list for coronary bypass surgery. *New Zealand Medical Journal* **110**(1037): 26–30.

Egbert, L.D., Battit, G.E., Welch, C.E. & Bartlett, M.K. (1964) Reduction of postoperative pain by encouragement and instruction of patients. *New England Journal of Medicine* **270**: 825–7.

Engleman, D., Adams, D., Bryne, J. *et al.* (1999) Impact of body mass index and albumin on morbidity and mortality after cardiac surgery. *Journal of Thoracic and Cardiovascular Surgery* **118**(5): 866–73.

Epstein, S.K., Faling, L.J., Daly, B.D. *et al.* (1993) Predicting complication after pulmonary resection: preoperative exercise testing vs multifactorial cardiopulmonary index. *Chest* **104**: 694–700.

Fitzsimons, D., Richardson, S. & Scott, M. (2000) Prospective study of clinical and func-tional status in patients awaiting coronary artery bypass surgery. *Coronary Health Care* **4**: 117–22.

Fletcher, C.M. (Chairman) (1960) Standardised questionnaire on respiratory symptom: a statement prepared and approved by the MRC committee on the aetiology of chronic bronchitis (MRC breathlessness score). *British Medical Journal* **2**: 1665s.

Galloway, S., Bubela, N., McKibbon, A., McCay, E. & Ross, E. (1993) Perceived information needs and effect of symptoms on activities after surgery for lung cancer. *Cancer Oncology Nurse* **3**: 116–19.

Gass, G.D. & Olsen, G.N. (1986) Preoperative pulmonary function testing to predict post-operative morbidity and mortality. *Chest* **89**: 127–35.

Ghosh, S. & Latimer, R.D. (1999) *Thoracic Anaesthesia: Principles and Practice*. Butterworth-Heinemann, Oxford.

Goldman, L. (1995) Cardiac risk in noncardiac surgery: an update. *Anaesthesia and Analgesia* **80**,: 810–20.

Goldman, L., Caldera, D., Nussbaum, S., Southwick, F., Krogtad, D. & Murray, B. (1977) Multifactorial index of cardiac risk in noncardiac surgical procedures. *New England Journal of Medicine* **297**: 845–50.

Goldstraw, P. (1987) Post-operative management of the thoracic surgical patient. In: Gothard, J.W.W. (ed.) *Thoracic Anaesthesia: Clinical anaesthesiology*. Baillière Tindall, London.

Hahnel, J., Mutschler, D., Huhn, W. *et al.* (1994) Endothelin, ACTH and cortisol plasma levels in patients undergoing aortocoronary bypass grafting. *Anaesthetist* **43**: 635–41.

Hammon, J.W. Jr, Stump, D.A., Kon, N.D. *et al.* (1997) Risk factors and solutions for the development of neurobehavioural changes after coronary artery bypass. *Annals of Thoracic Surgery* **63**: 1613–18.

Haydock, D. & Hill, G. (1987) Improved wound healing response in surgical patients receiving intravenous nutrition. *British Journal of Surgery* **74**: 320–23.

Hayward, J. (1975) *Information – A Prescription Against Pain*. Royal College of Nursing, London.

Helgeson, V. (1999) Applicability of cognitive adaptation theory to predicting adjustment to heart disease after coronary angioplasty. *Health Psychology* **18**(6): 561–9.

Helm, R., Gold, J., Rosengart, T., Zelano, J., Isom, O. & Krieger, K. (1993) Erythropoietin in cardiac surgery. *Journal of Cardiac Surgery* **8**(5): 579–606.

Hill, G. (1992) *Disorders of Nutrition and Metabolism in Clinical Surgery: Understanding and Management*. Churchill Livingstone, Edinburgh.

Hubbard, P., Muhlenkamp, A. & Brown, N. (1984) The relationship between social support and self-care practices. *Nursing Research* **33**: 266–9.

Jakob, H., Borneff-Lipp, M., Bach, A. *et al.* (2000) The endogenous pathway is a major route for deep sternal wound infection. *European Journal of Cardiothoracic Surgery* **17**(2): 1154–60.

Janssens, J., Pache, J. & Nicod, L. (1999) Physiological changes in respiratory function associated with ageing. *European Respiratory Journal* **13**(1): 197–205.

Jenkins, C.D., Stanton, B. & Jono, R.T. (1994) Quantifying and predicting recovery after surgery. *Psychosomatic Medicine* **56**: 203–12.

Jickling, J. & Graydon, J. (1997) The information needs at time of hospital discharge of male and female patients who have undergone coronary artery bypass grafting: a pilot study. *Heart and Lung* **26**(5): 350–57.

Jones, H.J.S. & deCossart, L. (1999) Risk scoring in surgical patients. *The British Journal of Surgery* **86**(2): 149–57.

Kearney, D.J., Lee, T.H., Reilly, J.J., DeCamp, M.M. & Sugarbaker, D.J. (1994) Assessment of operative risk in patients undergoing lung resection: importance of predicted pulmonary function. *Chest* **105**: 753–9.

Keene, A.R. & Cullen, D.J. (1983) Therapeutic intervention scoring system: update 1983. *Critical Care Medicine* **11**: 1–3.

Kiecolt-Glaser, J.K., Page, G.G., Marucha, P.T., MacCallum, R.C. & Glaser, R. (1998) Psychological influences on surgical recovery: perspectives from psychoneuro-immunology. *American Psychologist* **53**: 1209–18.

Kiecolt-Glaser, J.K., McGuire, L., Robles, T.F. & Glaser, R. (2002) Psychoneuroimmunology and psychosomatic medicine: back to the future. *Psychosomatic Medicine* **64**(1): 15–28.

King, K. (1985) Measurement of coping strategies, concerns and emotional response in patients undergoing coronary artery bypass grafting. *Heart and Lung* **14**(6): 579–93.

Kirschbaum, C. & Hellhammer, D.H. (1994) Salivary cortisol in psychoneuroendocrine research: recent developments and applications. *Psychoneuroendocrinology* **19**: 313–33.

Klopfenstein, C., Forster, A. & Van Gesel, E. (2000) Anesthetic assessment in an outpatient consultation clinic reduces preoperative anxiety. *Canadian Journal of Anaesthesia* **47**(6): 511–15.

Knaus, W.A., Draper, E.A., Wagner, D.P. & Zimmerman, J.E. (1985) APACHE II: a severity of disease classification system. *Critical Care Medicine* **13**: 818–29.

Koivula, M., Paunonen-Ilmonen, M., Tarkka, M., Tarkka, M. & Laippala, P. (2001) Gender differences and fears in patients awaiting coronary artery bypass grafting. *Journal of Clinical Nursing* **19**(4): 538–49.

Koltun, W.A., Bloomer, M., Tilberg, A.F. *et al.* (1996) Awake epidural anesthesia is associated with improved natural killer cell cytotoxicity and a reduced stress response. *American Journal of Surgery* **171**(1): 68–73.

Kroenke, K., Lawrence, V.A., Theroux, J.F. & Tuley, M.R. (1992) Operative risk in patients with severe obstructive pulmonary disease. *Archives & Internal Medicine* **152**: 967–71.

Lamberts, S.W.J., Bruining, H.A. & de Jong, F.H. (1997) Drug therapy: corticosteroid therapy in severe illness. *New England Journal of Medicine* **337**(18): 1285–92.

Lawrence, V., Dhanda, R., Hilsenbeck, S. & Page, C. (1996) Risk of pulmonary complications after elective abdominal surgery. *Chest* **110**: 744–50.

Lawrence, D., Valencia, O., Smith, E., Murday, A. & Treasure, T. (2000) Parsonnet score is a good predictor of the duration of intensive care unit stay following cardiac surgery. *Heart* **83**(4): 429–32.

Lazarus, R.S. & Folkman, S. (1984) *Stress, Appraisal and Coping*. Springer, New York.

Lefor, A. (1999) Perioperative management of the patient with cancer. *Chest* **115**(5): 165S–171S.

Lepzcyk, M., Raleigh, E.H. & Rowley, C. (1990) Timing of preoperative patient teaching. *Journal of Advanced Nursing* **15**(3): 300–306.

Lim, L.L.Y., Johnson, N.A., O'Connell, R.L. & Heller, R.F. (1998) Quality of life and later adverse health outcomes in patients with suspected heart attack. *Australian and New Zealand Journal of Public Health* **22**: 540–46.

Lindsay, G., Hinnie, J. & Gaw, A. (1995) Setting up a helpline on heart disease. *Nursing Standard* **10**(10): 27–30.

Lindsay, G., Smith, L., Hanlon, P. & Wheatley, D. (2001) The influence of general health status and social support on symptomatic outcome following coronary artery bypass grafting. *Heart* **85**(1): 80–86.

MacPherson, D.S. & Lofgren, R.P. (1994) Outpatient internal medicine preoperative evaluation: a randomised clinical trial. *Medical Care* **32**: 498–507.

Mangano, D. & Goldman, L. (1995) Current concepts: preoperative assessment of patients with known or suspected coronary disease. *New England Journal of Medicine* **333**(26): 1750–56.

Mark, J., Lockhart, L., McMeekan, K. & Isles, C. (1997) How well do we support our patients between angiography and bypass surgery? *Coronary Health Care* **1**: 18–21.

Matthews, K., Gump, B. & Owens, J. (2001) Chronic stress influences cardiovascular and neuroendocrine responses during acute stress and recovery, especially in men. *Health Psychology* **20**(6): 403–10.

McClave, S.A. & Snider, H.L. (1999) Preoperative issues in clinical nutrition. *Chest* **115**(5): 64S–70S.

McConachie, I. (2002) *Anaesthesia for the High Risk Patient*. Greenwich Medical Media, London.

McEwen, B.S. (1998) Seminars in medicine of the Beth Israel Deaconess Medical Centre: protective and damaging effects of stress mediators. *New England Journal of Medicine* **338**(3): 171–9.

McHugh, F., Lindsay, G., Hanlon, P. *et al.* (2001) Nurse led shared care for patients on the waiting list for coronary artery bypass surgery: a randomized controlled trial. *Heart* **86**(3): 317–23.

Melendez, J.A., Carlon, V. & Arslan, M.D. (1998) Cardiopulmonary risk index does not predict complications after thoracic surgery. *Chest* **114**(1): 69–75.

Mercuriali, F. & Inghilleri, G. (1998) Management of preoperative anaemia. *British Journal of Anaesthesia* **81**(Suppl. 1): 56–61.

Minowada, G. & Welch, W.I. (1995) Clinical implications of the stress response. *Journal of Clinical Investigation* **95**: 3–12.

Moore, S. (1995) A comparison of women's and men's symptoms during home recovery after coronary artery bypass surgery. *Heart and Lung* **24**(6): 495–501.

Moser, D. (1994) Social support and cardiac recovery. *Journal of Cardiovascular Nursing* **9**(1): 27–36.

Moser, D.K. & Dracup, K. (1995) Psychosocial recovery from a cardiac event: the influence of perceived control. *Heart and Lung* **24**: 273–80.

Mountain, C.F. (1997) Revisions in the international system for staging lung cancer. *Chest* **111**: 1710.

Newman, M.F., Kirchner, J.L., Phillips-Bute, B. *et al.* (2001) Longitudinal assessment of neurocognitive function after coronary artery bypass surgery. *New England Journal of Medicine* **344**(6): 395–402.

Paccagnella, A., Carlo, M., Caerno, G. *et al.* (1994) Cardiac cachexia: preoperative and postoperative nutrition management. *Journal of Parenteral and Enteral Nutrition* **18**(5): 409–16.

Papanicolaou, D.A., Wilder, R.L., Manolagas, S. & Chrousos, G.P. (1998) The pathophysiological roles of interleukin-6 in human disease. *Annals of Internal Medicine* **128**(2): 127–37.

Parsonnet, V., Dean, D. & Bernstein, A. (1989) A method of uniform stratification for evaluating the results of surgery in acquired adult heart disease. *Circulation* **79**(6)(Suppl. 1): 1–9.

Peters, M.L., Godaert, L.R. & Ballieux, R.E. (1998) Cardiovascular and endocrine responses to experimental stress: effects of mental effort and controlability. *Psychoneuroendocrinology* **23**: 1–17.

Pollock, R.E., Lotzova, E. & Standord, S.D. (1992) Surgical stress impairs natural killer cell programming of tumor for lysis in patients with sarcomas and other solid tumors. *Cancer* **70**: 2192–202.

Pollock, H.H.G., Street, M.K. & Boyd, O. (2000) Optimisation of the high risk surgical patient. *Surgery* **18**: 171–81.

Pons, J.M., Espinas, J.A., Borras, J.M., Moreno, V., Martin, I. & Granados, A. (1998) Cardiac surgical mortality: comparison among different additive risk-scoring models in a multicenter sample. *Archives of Surgery* **133**(10): 1053–7.

Rakoczy, M. (1997) The thoughts and feelings of patients in the waiting period prior to cardiac surgery: a descriptive study. *Heart and Lung* **6**(2): 280–87.

Rennotte, M.T., Baele, P., Aubert, G. & Rodenstein, D. (1995) Nasal continuous positive airway pressure in the perioperative management of patients with obstructive sleep apnoea submitted to surgery. *Chest* **107**(2): 367–74.

Riley, J. (1995) Fast track cardiac care. *Nursing Standard* **9**(49): 55–6.

Rosenberg, J. & Kehlet, H. (1991) Post-operative episodic oxygen desaturation in the sleep apnoea syndrome. *Acta Anaesthesiologica Scandinavica* **35**(4): 368–9.

Royal College of Physicians and Royal College of Psychiatrists (1995) *The Psychological Care of Medical Patients*. Royal College of Physicians and Royal College of Psychiatrists, London.

Ryhanen, P., Huttunen, K. & Ilonen, J. (1984) Natural killer cell activity after open heart surgery. *Acta Anaesthesiologica Scandinavica* **28**: 490–92.

Schmiesing, C.A. & Fischer, P. (2001) The preoperative assessment of the cancer patient. *Current Opinion in Anaesthesiology* **14**(6): 721–9.

Selnes, O.A., Goldsborough, M.A., Borawicz, L.M. & McKhann, G.M. (1999) Neurobehavioural sequelae of cardiopulmonary bypass. *Lancet* **353**: 1601–6.

Selye, H. (1956) *The Stress of Life.* McGraw-Hill, New York.

Shaw, C. (1999) A framework for the study of coping, illness behavior and outcomes. *Journal of Advanced Nursing* **29**(5): 1246–55.

Shuldham, C. (1999) A review of the impact of pre-operative education on recovery from surgery. *International Journal of Nursing Studies* **36**(2): 171–7. (This article provides a useful review of experimental studies of preoperative education.)

Smyth, J., Ockenfels, C.M., Porter, L., Kirschbaum, C., Hellhammer, D.H. & Stone, A.A. (1998) Stressors and mood measured on a momentary basis are associated with salivary cortisol secretion. *Psychoneuroendocrinology* **23**: 353–70.

Teo, K., Spoor, M., Pressey, T. *et al.* (1998) Impact of managed waiting for coronary artery bypass graft surgery on patient perceived quality of life. *Circulation* **98**(19S): 29II–33II.

Thoits, P.A. (1995) Stress, coping and social support processes: Where are we? What next? *Journal of Health and Social Behaviour* (Extra Issue): 53–79.

Thomas, R., Polanski, P., Gorden, W. & Just-Viera, S. (1995) Early complications and longterm survival in severely obese patients. *The American Surgeon* **61**(11): 949–63.

Tonnesen, E., Brinklov, M., Christensen, N.J., Olesen, A.S. & Madsen, T. (1987) Natural killer cell activity and lymphocyte function during and after coronary artery bypass grafting in relation to the endocrine stress response. *Anaesthesiology* **67**: 526–33.

Warner, D.O., Warner, M.A., Barnes, R.D. *et al.* (1996) Perioperative respiratory complications in patients with asthma. *Anaesthesiology* **85**: 460–67.

Wilson-Barnett, J. (1979) *Stress in Hospital: Patient's Psychological Reactions to Illness and Healthcare.* Churchill Livingstone, Edinburgh.

Wisser, W., Klepetko, W., Senbaklavaci, O. *et al.* (1998) Chronic hypercapnia should not exclude patients from lung volume reduction surgery. *European Journal of Cardiothoracic Surgery* **14**(2): 107–12.

Wong, J. & Wong, S. (1985) A randomized controlled trial of a new approach to preoperative teaching and patient compliance. *International Journal of Nursing Studies* **22**(2): 105–15.

Zacharias, A. & Habib, R. (1996) Factors predisposing to median sternotomy complications: deep versus superficial infection. *Chest* **110**: 1173–8.

Zigmund, A.S. & Snaith, R.P. (1983) The hospital anxiety and depression scale. *Acta Psychiatrica Scandinavica* **67**: 361–70.

Further reading

Bickley, L.S. & Szilagyi, P.G. (2000) *Bates' Guide to Physical Examination and History Taking.* Lippincott Williams & Wilkins, Philadelphia, USA.

Jarvis, C. (2003) *Pocket Companion for Physical Examination and Health Assessment.* W.B. Saunders, Philadelphia, USA.

McHugh, F., Hankey, C. & Belcher, P.R. (2000) The management of patients on the waiting list for coronary artery bypass grafting: a case study. *Coronary Health Care* **4**: 146–51.

Sotile, W.M. (1996) *Psychosocial Interventions for Cardiopulmonary Patients: A Guide for Health Professionals.* Human Kinetics, Leeds.

Intra-operative Issues

Many factors may contribute to the development of post-operative complications, not least the events which occur during the time the patient is in the operating room, including those related to anaesthesia and the surgical techniques employed. An understanding of these issues will help the nurse to appreciate just how vulnerable the patient is post-operatively. Indeed, it could be argued that the intra-operative period may have the most significant impact on post-operative outcome.

The anaesthetic

Anaesthetists and surgeons are developing new techniques all the time which minimise the surgical stress response. Pre-medication protocols will probably include benzodiazepines, butyrophenes, opiates and anticholinergics. An important aim is to reduce anxiety thus decreasing sympathetic arousal. Drugs which may be given initially include the benzodiazepines (e.g. midazolam, lorazepam and diazepam) and some may act as amnesic agents. An anticholinergic such as atropine or scopolamine is frequently used to reduce secretions and will facilitate instrumentation of the airways and prevent vomiting. Anticholinergics, however, reduce vagal activity to the heart, and caution needs to be exercised when using atropine in patients with a history of coronary heart disease because of the associated tachycardia and reduced coronary perfusion. Although scopolamine can result in post-operative delirium in the elderly (Kolker 1997), it does have more sedating and anti-emetic properties than atropine and causes less tachycardia.

For induction, fentanyl, an opiate, is a common agent as it is lipid soluble, acts rapidly and tends to have fewer cardiovascular effects. An alternative is propofol. A muscle relaxant is necessary and these agents work at the neuromuscular junction of skeletal muscle. Muscle contraction usually occurs due to stimulation of nicotinic receptors by acetylcholine on the motor end plate. This mechanism can be altered by giving a non-depolarising drug which competes with acetylcholine at the receptor site. Examples of non-depolarising agents used during long surgical procedures are pancuronium and vecuronium which tends to cause less tachycardia and hypertension. For more minor procedures, a shorter-acting depolarising agent such as succinylcholine which causes fasciculation of muscle units is used. When these agents are used, paralysis of muscles occurs and the patient must be intubated and ventilated. Non-depolarising agents are reversed by the administration of neostigmine, although this can precipitate atrioventricular nodal disorders (Jarpe 1992).

Propofol is often used together with fentanyl, particularly in fast-track patients, as it has been found to give a lower incidence of tachycardia and hypertension and has a small metabolic suppressant effect which is beneficial in patients with myocardial ischaemia. Once propofol is discontinued, extubation may take place within a much shorter time period.

Once the patient has been successfully intubated then maintenance of anaesthesia is achieved by intravenous drugs such as propofol, fentanyl or midazolam and inhaled isoflurane and oxygen with nitrous oxide or air. Isoflurane may be preferred because of its tendency not to cause ventricular dysrhythmias and this may benefit patients who have been receiving aminophylline and/or β-adrenergic agonists. During surgery, although the patient is unconscious the physiological response to painful stimuli can still be activated. Intra-operative analgesia will reduce sympathetic arousal in response to pain, minimise the risk of myocardial ischaemia and dysrhythmias and also reduce the neuroendocrine surgical stress response. Because the stress response in major surgery results in a catabolic hypermetabolic state there is increased oxygen consumption which can be detrimental. Analgesia is necessary, therefore, throughout the surgical procedure and an intravenous opiate such as fentanyl is administered.

During cardiothoracic surgery bronchoconstriction may occur because of neurohormonal and local mediator release and this is often associated with pulmonary disease. Fentanyl is therefore preferable to morphine as there is less risk of histamine release with hypotension (Barr & Donner 1995). Additional opioids which do not result in histamine release are sufentanil, alfentanil and remifentanil. An epidural cannula is often inserted for thoracic surgery and this may be used to administer either opioids alone or with a local anaesthetic such as bupivacaine. There is work to suggest that the epidural may be more effective when placed before surgery begins.

The choice and combination of pharmacological agents is crucial. For example, in cardiac surgery one important objective is to control haemodynamic changes which occur during surgery, often necessitating the use of either vasopressors for hypotension or β-blockade for tachycardia and hypertension. It has been shown, therefore, that the interaction of pre-medication, induction agent and relaxant is important.

During cardiac and thoracic surgery, oxygen delivery to the tissues must still be ensured and the steps taken to achieve this goal will vary between the two types of surgery. The next two sections outline the techniques used in cardiac and thoracic surgery and the major factors which can compromise cardiopulmonary status.

Cardiac surgery

Revascularisation

Coronary artery bypass surgery is not normally the first treatment option for coronary heart disease. Risk reduction through lifestyle modification, together with drug therapy to relieve angina and reduce the risk of heart failure, is the first line of treatment. However, when these fail to control symptoms, intervention through percutaneous transluminal angioplasty (PCTA) and stent or coronary artery bypass grafting (CABG) should be considered. Generally, the presence of left main stem disease, or three-vessel disease with moderately impaired left ventricular function, are clear indicators for cardiac surgery (Pillai & Wright 1999; Abrahamov *et al.* 2000). Additionally, when there is diffuse vessel disease, more frequently found in the diabetic population, coronary artery bypass surgery is more likely. Surgery however, is not without risk and the overall operative morbidity is around 2% with increased mortality in the older age group, women, or those with co-morbidity (Abrahamov *et al.* 2000). When successful, surgery is associated with good long-term survival to almost 20 years (Bradshaw *et al.* 2002).

The more common conduits used for CABG include the saphenous vein, internal mammary artery and radial artery (see Fig. 5.1). Less commonly used are the gastro-epiploic, the ulnar or the inferior epigastric arteries. Where possible, the internal mammary artery (IMA) is used, largely due to its longer patency rate of around 10 years (Taggart 2002). The IMA appears to be more resistant to atheroma formation over native coronary arteries and vein grafts, owing to the greater ability of the endothelium to influence vasculature tone, provide a non-thrombogenic surface and respond to the inflammatory process (De Jaegere & Suyker 2002). However, the use of the IMA may lead to various complications, such as delayed sternal wound healing, especially in the diabetic population, and increased respiratory complications due largely to the opening of the pleura and the concomitant increase in pain. The use of the bilateral internal mammary artery (BIMA), although of clear benefit, is reserved for carefully selected patients and usually avoided in those with uncontrolled diabetes, chronic respiratory conditions, the obese and heavy smokers. When BIMA grafting is anticipated, the increase in risk should be recognised and measures taken to prevent post-operative respiratory and wound complications.

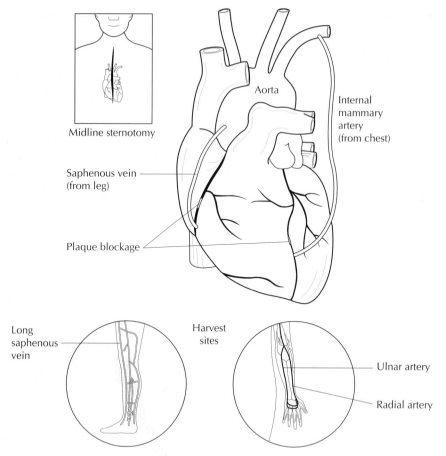

Midline sternotomy

Aorta

Internal mammary artery (from chest)

Saphenous vein (from leg)

Plaque blockage

Long saphenous vein

Harvest sites

Ulnar artery

Radial artery

Fig. 5.1   Location of incisions and graft sites for coronary revascularisation. From Mathews (2002), with permission.

Minimally invasive coronary artery surgery (MICS)

Techniques to make coronary artery bypass surgery less invasive include minimal access incision sites, eliminating the need for cardiopulmonary bypass (CPB) and avoiding manipulation of the aorta.

When the aim is to avoid a median sternotomy, a small incision of around 10 cm is made in the anterior thoracotomy wall. This smaller incision may reduce complications in terms of wound and chest infection although the thorocotomy site may be more painful than the traditional sternotomy (Lichtenberg *et al.* 2000; Ng *et al.* 2000). An additional advantage of the small incision site is that any 'redo' operation can be performed through a median sternotomy as virgin territory. However, a median sternotomy without CPB is the more frequently used procedure, enhancing visualisation and access to all heart vessels, while avoiding the need for CPB.

These less invasive techniques appear to reduce the morbidity and mortality associated with cardiac surgery, may reduce the length of hospital stay and may lead to the earlier resumption of work and social activities (Jansen *et al.* 1998).

However, they also have their limitations and the risk is further influenced by the surgeon's experience, access, exposure and visualisation of the coronary vessels, haemodynamic support and anastomosis.

Endoscopic coronary artery surgery, using a mini-sternotomy and port access technique is developing, with the surgeon performing CABG or valve surgery through a small incision with videoscopic assistance. This is likely to confer major benefit to the patient with regard to their post-operative course and outcome.

Transmyocardial laser revascularisation has received brief interest, with the concept based on the reptilian circulation and the idea that the creation of transmural channels between the myocardium and the ventricular cavity will improve perfusion. The exact science behind this is unclear, although channels may allow oxygenated blood from the cavity to seep into the heart muscle. Others believe that new channels close over in time but stimulate angiogenesis (Hayden 1998). This form of surgery is still experimental and not widely used either in Europe or in the USA.

Valvular heart disease

Surgery for valvular heart disease may include valve repair or replacement and recent years have seen a profusion of valves available on the market (see Fig. 5.2). The choice of valve may depend upon the age of the patient, their religion, or the long-term need for anticoagulation. Although the surgeon makes the choice of valve, it is useful for the nurse to have some knowledge of the factors that may influence this choice (see Table 5.1)

For the women of childbearing age, valve disease should be treated before a planned pregnancy, preferably by balloon valvuloplasty or valve repair. Pregnancy may possibly accelerate the degeneration of the valve (Bloomfield 2002), and a mechanical valve will necessitate anticoagulation with the inevitable risk to both the mother and baby. Warfarin crosses the placenta barrier where it may cause spontaneous abortion, stillbirth or premature birth. However, heparin does not cross the placenta barrier and may be a safer drug for the fetus, although possibly increases the risk of thromboembolism. The difficulty in satisfactorily managing pregnancy in a patient with a mechanical valve prosthesis requires that they be treated in a specialist unit.

Currently, valve replacement requires a median sternotomy and CPB. However, as techniques develop a smaller incision or port access is likely to be more common (De Amicis *et al.* 1997). More widespread use of minimally invasive valve replacement is likely to offer particular benefit to the obese, the diabetic or those with chronic lung disease.

Aortic dissection

Widely used as a classification system, the Stanford classification of aortic dissection identifies type A as a dissection of the aorta involving the ascending aorta whereas type B extends to the descending thoracic aorta, distal to the left subclavian artery and is therefore outside the remit of this text.

Table 5.1 Types of heart valve

Type of valve	Description	Special issues
Mechanical valves	**Used in the younger patient or in those already receiving anticoagulation therapy**	
Ball valve	Starr–Edwards: silastic ball which moves into the sewing ring when closed and into the cage when open	Original design has been modified and is still in use today Lifelong anticoagulation required. Target INR 3.0–4.5
Disc valve	Bjork–Shiley: graphite disc, coated with carbon. This disc tilts to open and close Disc valves still produced by other manufacturers	Bjork–Shiley valve is no longer manufactured Lifelong anticoagulation required. Target INR 3.0–4.5
Bileaflet valve	The St Jude valve is the most popular in current use. This valve has two semicircular leaflets that open and close	Lifelong anticoagulation required, although possibly with lower intensity warfarin therapy (maintaining an INR 2.5–3.0 for aortic replacement and 3.0–3.5 for mitral valve replacement) Long-term durability of the valve has been reported
Biological valve	**Used in the elderly or to avoid long-term anticoagulation (expected to last approximately 10 years)**	
Autologous valve; patients own tissue used to create a valve (fascia lata or pericardium)	Infrequently used today	

Autograft; patients own valve placed into another position within the heart (e.g. pulmonary valve used in the aortic position)	Designed by Donald Ross and termed the Ross procedure. The pulmonary valve is used to replace a diseased aortic valve. The pulmonary valve is replaced by a pulmonary homograft. This procedure is of particular use in children as the translocated pulmonary trunk can grow with the child's development	Late problems associated with failure of the pulmonary homograft. The procedure is a double valve replacement and so requires a lengthy anaesthetic
Homograft: valve transplanted from a human cadaver heart	The cadaver heart valve is sterilised and stored. They can be used either as a fresh valve or from frozen	Longer period of time on cardiopulmonary bypass. Useful in aortic dissection affecting the aortic root
Xenograft: valve transplanted from another animal (e.g. pig) or manufactured from bovine tissue such as the pericardium	These valves are sterilised and stored for use	Religious or cultural reasons may make the use of an animal valve inappropriate

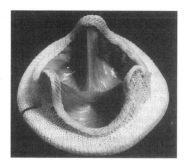
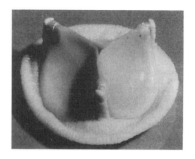
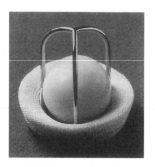
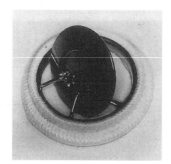
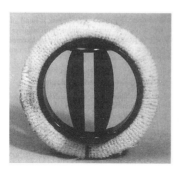

Fig. 5.2   Examples of heart valves. Reprinted from Julian (1989), with permission from Elsevier Science.

Treatment of a type A dissection requires surgical repair of the aorta. The aim of surgical treatment is to remove and replace the existing aortic segment where the dissection originates, rather than remove the entire dissecting aortic tissue. Where the dissection extends to the coronary arteries or aortic valve, surgery is complicated by reimplantation of the coronary arteries and aortic valve replacement.

The operation is generally performed as an emergency, through a median sternotomy and using CPB with right atrial and femoral artery cannulation. More recently there has been interest in the use of an endovascular stent. Similar to those used in the coronary arteries, the stent is inserted into the aorta and lies over the area of aneurysm or dissection, thereby avoiding the need for major surgery. Although there are promising reports of early success, long-term follow-up data is not yet available (Khan & Nair 2002).

Occasionally, the dissection may extend to the aortic valve and in these circumstances aortic valve replacement will also be required. The use of a homograft, enabling the entire aortic root to be replaced, is now the operation of choice. The operative mortality for this procedure is estimated at 5–11%.

Cardiopulmonary bypass

Traditionally, cardiac surgery has been undertaken on a heart that is still and bloodless. The body's oxygen requirements are reduced and the organs and tissues oxygenated through an extracorporeal circulation or cardiopulmonary bypass. This means that the lungs can be deflated to maximise visualisation of the operative site and allows temporary disruption to the circulatory system for the period of surgery, without causing global ischaemia.

Following a median sternotomy, CPB is commenced. The right atrium is cannulated and blood diverted from the right side of the heart into the CPB machine. A series of roller pumps circulates the blood past a membrane oxygenator and returns it to the systemic circulation via an aortic cannula (Fig. 5.3). Once blood is circulating through the CPB, the body temperature is rapidly reduced. A clamp is then placed across the aorta between the heart and the aortic cannula to ensure that blood from the bypass machine does not flow into the heart, but forwards into the systemic circulation.

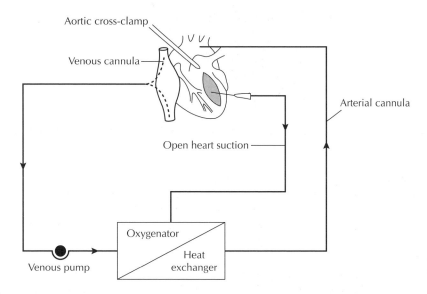

Fig. 5.3 Cardiopulmonary bypass.

For effective CPB the following issues are important:

- Blood must be heparinised to prevent clotting in the extracorporeal circulation. An activated clotting time of around 450 s (normal 90–120 s) should be maintained. Heparinisation is reversed at the end of surgery with protamine sulphate.
- Blood is haemodiluted with a crystalloid solution to aid movement through the CPB and this contributes to the low haematocrit and low blood pressure frequently seen in the immediate post-operative period.
- Blood must be oxygenated before it is returned to the systemic circulation. This is achieved by the blood flowing past a membrane oxygenator, which not only oxygenates the blood but also removes carbon dioxide.

During CPB, blood comes into contact with a foreign surface that activates the complement system and the inflammatory response. Oxygen free radicals and pro-inflammatory cytokines are activated and may contribute to the myocardial stunning, respiratory distress syndrome, renal failure, neurological injury and pancreatitis, sometimes observed in the post-operative period (De Jaegere & Suyker 2002) (see Table 5.2). To prevent this, evolving practice includes avoiding CPB and hypothermia, changes in operative techniques, and pharmacological agents that may reduce heart damage from ischaemia.

In addition to the bloodless field necessary for traditional cardiac surgery, the heart needs to remain still to allow the surgeon to operate. This can be achieved through two principal methods: cross-clamp with fibrillation and cardioplegia.

Cross-clamp and fibrillation

Cross-clamp and fibrillation is appropriate for CABG when the surgeon only requires the heart to be still during the distal anastomosis when the graft is sewn to the heart tissue itself. For this procedure, the body is cooled so that the oxygen requirement is reduced and the heart protected from ischaemic injury. Ventricular fibrillation is induced by using a low-voltage current, reducing the myocardial oxygen requirement still further. Once the distal anastomosis is complete, the cross-clamp is removed and blood flows into the heart chambers. Another low-voltage DC shock restores the heart to sinus rhythm. This process can be repeated for each distal anastomosis and is used successfully when the period of cross-clamp and fibrillation is no longer than 15 minutes each time and with a total cross-clamp period of under 60 minutes. As the time required to perform the distal anastomosis cannot reliably be predicted, many surgeons prefer to use a cardioplegic solution to arrest the heart.

Cardioplegia

Another method to protect the heart during CPB is to infuse a cardioplegic solution which is high in potassium (usually 15–30 mmol/l). Intracellular potas-

Table 5.2 Complications of cardiopulmonary bypass

Organ/system	Problem	Effect	Post-operative consequence
Cardiovascular	Myocardial ischaemia	Myocardial stunning	Depressed myocardial function Arrhythmia formation
	Hypothermia	Increased blood viscosity	Labile blood pressure
	Haemodilution	Decreased blood viscosity Diuresis	Low blood pressure Hypokalaemia
	Decreased baroreceptor activity	Vasoconstriction	Labile blood pressure
	Heparinisation	Prolonged bleeding time	Risk of bleeding
	Platelet damage	Decreased platelet count	Risk of bleeding
Pulmonary	Deflated lungs	Reduced surfactant production	Atelectasis
	Inflammatory response	Increased capillary leakage	Respiratory distress syndrome
Renal	Decreased renal blood flow	Kidney dysfunction	Acute renal failure
Neurological	Risk of air embolism or disruption of calcified plaque	Neurological/cognitive dysfunction	Cerebrovascular accident Behavioural changes Post-pump psychosis
Systemic inflammatory response	Increased catecholamine secretion	Vasoconstriction	Hypertension
	Increased cytokine release	Increased glycogenesis	Elevated blood glucose levels
		Increased capillary permeability	'Pump lung syndrome'

sium will no longer diffuse out of the cell, the resting membrane potential will rise and the cell will remain in a continuous state of partial depolarisation, rendering it motionless. Following aortic cross-clamping the cardioplegic solution is infused under pressure into the aorta or coronary sinus, where it will flow down the coronary arteries. The solution can be reinfused as required throughout the operation.

Debate continues regarding the choice of cardioplegic solution, and the variety of solutions indicates that there is no clear advantage of any one. The choice of solution remains the province of the operating surgeon. However, for the nurse caring for the patient in the post-operative period, differences in post-operative care will be noted and so this subject warrants a brief discussion here.

- **Cold crystalloid cardioplegia:** potassium is added to a hyperosmolar solution, usually Ringer's lactate. The cold temperature (15–20°C) and high potassium concentration will lead to ventricular standstill and a motionless operative field, thereby reducing myocardial oxygen consumption. However, the cold crystalloid cardioplegia also alters platelet function, impairs calcium influx and leads to myocardial cell oedema. Crystalloid solutions also deplete adenosine triphosphate stores.
- **Blood cardioplegia:** blood is mixed with the cardioplegic solution and by providing oxygen, is able to supply the heart tissues with an energy source. Through maintaining an oncotic pressure, less myocardial oedema develops, and less reperfusion injury occurs. In high-risk patients, the use of blood may enhance myocardial protection and decrease the development of life-threatening arrhythmias (Ibrahim *et al.* 1999), leading to a more stable post-operative period. However, this form of cardioplegia is more costly and takes longer to prepare and is not established for routine practice.

Reperfusion

Although frequently associated with the post-MI phase of recovery, reperfusion can occur whenever there has been a transient disruption to blood flow to the intrathoracic organs. With cardiac surgery, this may occur during aortic cross-clamping. A brief period of no perfusion followed by reperfusion will lead to reperfusion injury; leucocyte infiltration, thrombosis, oedema and vaso-constriction (Wang & Pinsky 2000). Furthermore, as oxygen levels rise, reactive oxidative stress (ROS) can be provoked and injures the endothelium. Normal vasoactive substances are altered, in particular nitric oxide secretion, and vaso-constriction becomes predominant, compounding the situation. Reperfusion injury is characterised by arrhythmias and haemodynamic changes. Pharmacological agents that alter the functioning of the cellular pumps and the influx of sodium may well prove beneficial in preventing reperfusion injury.

Ischaemic preconditioning

This phenomenon appears to suggest that brief periods of ischaemia may reduce the extent of myocardial ischaemic damage and so provide cardio-protection. This has been observed at the time of angioplasty, when greater changes are seen in the ST segment on the first balloon inflation over subsequent inflations. Brief periods of ischaemia appear to slow the rate of ATP depletion in subsequent ischaemic episodes and it would appear that ischaemic preconditioning may also offer benefit to the person undergoing cardiac surgery. Recent work has centred around the use of pharmacological agents prior to and/or during angioplasty or cardiac surgery or in patients with unstable angina (Keffelmann *et al.* 2000). By altering the gated channel action of the myocardial cell, they may prevent ischaemic changes and the rise in intracellular calcium. Intermittent reperfusion may also be beneficial by flushing out catabolites that have accumulated during the period of ischaemia and so prevent reperfusion injury and myocardial stunning.

Beating heart surgery

As the coronary arteries run epicardially across the heart, they can be operated on without opening the heart. Consequently, the heart does not have to be a bloodless field and the necessity for CPB is reduced. To maintain a motionless operating field, a device known as an octopus can be used to stabilise and immobilise a portion of the heart tissue during the anastomosis on the target vessel (Fig. 5.4). One such device uses two suction posts applying about $-400\,mmHg$ suction to the heart, and can be repositioned around the heart as required. As these stabilisers force the heart tissue downwards, they cause a temporary decrease in cardiac output and stroke volume, which requires more intensive intra-operative haemodynamic monitoring. Consequently, during beating heart surgery it is standard practice to insert a pulmonary artery catheter to measure haemodynamic parameters.

Ischaemia management is particularly important during beating heart surgery. To reduce myocardial oxygen consumption, the heart rate should be slowed with pharmacological agents and the myocardial oxygen supply maximised through

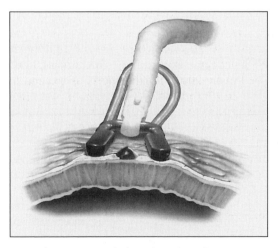

Fig. 5.4 Octopus. From Edgerton & Michelson (2000), with permission.

the use of nitrates and afterload reduction. Transoesophageal echocardiography is used continuously during the procedure to assess heart wall motion. Without the use of CPB, the lungs must remain ventilated. However, to maximise visualisation of the operative field, single lung ventilation with a double lumen endotracheal tube is used. If at any point there is evidence that the ischaemia is not tolerated, the surgeon may choose to convert to conventional surgery and CPB.

There are various advantages to the development of beating heart, or off-pump, surgery and these are outlined in Table 5.3. One of the main advantages rests with the reduction in the physiological consequences associated with CPB itself. Through eliminating some of these consequences, the risk of undergoing cardiac surgery to patients, particularly those at high risk, is reduced.

Table 5.3   Beating heart surgery

Advantages
- Avoids physiological consequences of CPB
- Avoids aortic cross-clamp

Indications
- Severely calcified aorta
- Renal disease
- Pulmonary disease
- Previous CVA
- Diffuse peripheral vascular disease
- High operative risk from conventional surgery

Contra-indications
- Deep intramyocardial vessels
- Small distal vessels
- Poor conduit
- Haemodynamic instability
- Acute myocardial infarction
- Cardiogenic shock

Thoracic surgery

For thoracic surgery it is often necessary to collapse the uppermost lung (non-ventilated), during the procedure while the dependent lung is ventilated. In the UK it is usual to use a double lumen endobronchial tube to facilitate one-lung surgery (see Fig. 5.5). It was the Swedish surgeon Carlen who, in 1948, developed the double lumen tube which was a breakthrough in thoracic surgery. Robershaw, a British surgeon, later developed a tube with a larger lumen offering less resistance (Ghosh & Latimer 1999). These tubes are available in different sizes and can be either right or left sided. Where the lung is being resected the tube is usually placed in the lung which is not being operated on. Although initial insertion is assisted by the use of a laryngoscope, the rest of the manoeuvre is relatively blind and the skill of an experienced anaesthetist is crucial. Placement of

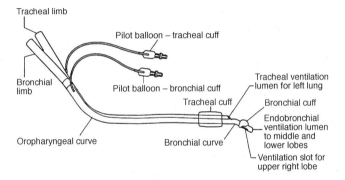

Fig. 5.5 Basic pattern of a modern right-sided double-lumen endobronchial tube. From Gothard (1993), with permission.

the tube is checked by fibre-optic bronchoscopy. The tube allows the anaesthetist to control the distribution of ventilation, allows surgical access to structures on the operated side and prevents contamination of the lower lung.

Position

Although thoracic surgery may be performed through a median sternotomy, many surgeons will enter the thorax through a posterolateral incision. For this the patient is placed in the lateral decubitus position as illustrated in Fig 5.6. Great care is taken to avoid injury, but even so the patient will experience some musculo-skeletal discomfort post-operatively due to the prolonged length of time in this position. This discomfort can be quite extreme if there is a history of musculo-skeletal problems. There are many thoracic surgical procedures which are performed and Table 5.4 outlines some of these.

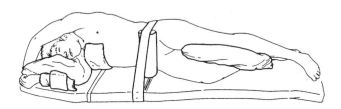

Fig. 5.6 The lateral thoracotomy position. From Gothard (1993), with permission.

The length of the skin incision extending from beneath the breast to approximately 3 cm beneath the scapula and the spine, and the incision of muscle layers (trapezius, latissimus and serratus muscles) which are divided with large retractors, contributes to the severe pain experienced following thoracotomy. The thoracic cavity is approached through the fifth or sixth intercostal space. In some patients where pulmonary status is compromised, performing a muscle-sparing incision where the muscles are retracted but not divided may reduce pain, disability and hypoventilation post-operatively (Hazelrigg *et al.* 1991). For patients

Table 5.4 Examples of thoracic surgical procedures

(a) Specific procedures

Location	Procedure	Description	Indications	Intra-operative issues	Special consideration
Surgery on the lung	Wedge resection	Resection of lung tissue with tumour irrespective of bronchopulmonary anatomy	Benign/malignant lesions which are localised and discrete (<3 cm dia.)	Procedure usually short often using only endotracheal intubation	Bleeding may be significant. Two chest drains used to remove blood and air from pleural space. Air leak usual. Suction up to 20 cm/H_2O usually applied
	Segmentectomy	Resection of discrete bronchopulmonary segment with blunt dissection	Used in poor-risk patients with limited pulmonary reserve	May be VATS procedure One lung ventilation may be used with double lumen tube	Avoid clamping of drains to reduce risk of tension pneumothorax
	Lobectomy	Removal of a lobe	Malignant/benign tumours Infection e.g. bronchiectasis tuberculosis and fungal infection		Two chest drains to underwater seal system – left open often with suction. Air leak usual
	Pneumonectomy	Removal of one lung	Usually for primary carcinoma or because of infection, e.g. tuberculosis	One lung ventilation with double lumen tube	Drains not clamped One drain may be inserted but left clamped. Unclamped for 1 min each hour. **No suction**

Surgery on the pleura, diaphragm and chest wall	Pleurectomy	Parietal pleura stripped except from diaphragmatic surface	For spontaneous pneumothoraces or secondary pneumothoraces following: COPD Cystic fibrosis Tuberculosis and lung cancer	Small thoracotomy incision (postero-lateral) or VATS Lung blebs and air leaks corrected	Chest drains inserted and suction applied. Very painful. Administer effective analgesia with IV opioids or epidural
	Pleurodesis	Pleural abrasion Technique used to initiate inflammatory reaction promoting pleural adhesion		Small thoracotomy incision or VATS often performed. Physical pleurodesis involves abrasion of pleural tissue with gauze. Chemical pleurodesis uses iodised talc	
	Decortication	Surgical removal of thick fibrous layer of tissue from pleural surface	Usually as a result of empyema or haemothorax and removal allows expansion and better chest movement on affected side	Small thoracotomy incision – usually posterolateral. A double lumen tube may be necessary particularly if there is a bronchopleural fistula	Chest drains inserted. Air leaks and bleeding common. The condition of the patient is usually poor often with chronic sepsis
Surgery on oesophagus	E.g. oesophagectomy	Resection with anastomosis	Removal of tumour usually in middle and lower third of oesophagus	Different techniques possible involving thoraco-abdominal/supine abdominal/laparotomy approaches Double lumen tube/one lung anaesthesia Various anastomoses and bypasses may be performed, e.g. oesophagogastrectomy	Short period of post-operative ventilation usual. Care taken to prevent aspiration of gastrointestinal contents

Contd

Table 5.4 *Contd*

(b) Other surgical procedures

Location	Description	Indications	Intra-operative issues	Special considerations
Lung transplant	Single lung transplantation (most common) Bilateral sequential transplantation, i.e. 2 single-lung transplants at the same time Heart–lung transplantation (decreasing) Transplantation of lobe(s) from live donor (usually in cystic fibrosis)	E.g. emphysema (α_1 anti-trypsin deficiency), interstitial lung disease, cystic fibrosis, primary pulmonary hypertension. Patients should have advanced lung disease unresponsive to other therapy, be relatively mobile but functionally disabled and free of significant cardiac, renal and hepatic impairment	Single lung with single-lung ventilation (usually without CPB) via posterolateral incision Bilateral – using transverse thoracosternotomy approach Live donor transplantation involves transplanting lower lobes from two donors	Lifelong immunosuppression Complications include primary graft failure anastomotic breakdown/stenosis, infection, acute/chronic rejection, bronchiolitis obliterans (Arcasoy & Kotloff 1999)
Lung volume reduction	Excision of 20–30% of the volume from each lung via median sternotomy	Severe emphysema where removing lung volume improves elastic recoil and reduces work of breathing High risk of death in patients with very low FEV_1 or gas transfer factor	One-lung surgery using double lumen tube. Median sternotomy usually performed and following volume reduction lung tissue stapled for example with bovine pericardial strips	Chest drains inserted with or without suction (two each side – reduced suction at $-10\,cm\,H_2O$). Air leaks can be problematical. Sternal dehiscence possible IV opioids avoided
Video-assisted thoracoscopic surgery (VATS)	Less invasive than open thoracotomy Series of ports used for instrumentation	Surgery such as pleurectomy, biopsy, pleurodesis and lung volume reduction	One-lung surgery with double lumen tube. The upper lung deflated prior to access ports and introduction of telescopes (Plummer et al. 1998)	Pain may be less in some instances although not for others, e.g. pleurectomy Chest drain inserted

Mediastinal surgery	Thymectomy	Results in clinical improvement in patients with myasthenia gravis	Various approaches – sternal/cervical	Chest drainage postoperatively Mediastinal drain
	Resection of mediastinal tumours	Primary neoplasms and cysts Two-thirds are benign (Strollo et al. 1997)	Median sternotomy Posterolateral thoracotomy	
Interventional bronchoscopy	Rigid/flexible bronchoscope used. Often for obstruction of trachea and main bronchi particularly where in advanced disease surgical resection is impossible	Primarily palliative, e.g. endoluminal airway obstruction Stenting for extrinsic airway compression Relief of symptoms caused by pleural effusions	Such interventional work often performed by experienced respiratory physicians. Laser ablation of central tumours. Neodymium:yttrium–aluminium–garnet (Nd:YAG) laser allows deep tissue penetration Endobronchial stent insertion Cryotherapy and electrocautery may be used for distal lesions Endobronchial brachytherapy (radiation source implanted)	Worsening haemodynamic and pulmonary status may be indicative of possible complications including: haemorrhage pneumothorax (Seijo & Sterman 2001)

who require oesophageal surgery the approach is often through the left hemi-thorax while lying on the right side.

The positioning during thoracic surgery can result in marked changes in ventilation perfusion relationships producing hypoxaemia which extends into the post-operative period. It is important to remember that these relationships are largely determined by gravitational forces. Although the upper lung is not ventilated it still receives pulmonary blood flow from the right ventricle and this results in significant right to left intra-pulmonary shunting during surgery. In addition, small areas of the lower lung collapse because of compression and a marked fall in the functional residual volume (Strandberg *et al.* 1986). Also contributing to collapse will be pooling of secretions which occurs in the airways during general anaesthesia. This problem is compounded if the ventilated lung is already impaired due to pulmonary disease, in which case severe arterial hypoxaemia may result, hence the importance of careful pre-operative evaluation of pulmonary function.

The preferential distribution of blood through the lower lung also contributes to a right to left shunt during surgery as the lower lung is less compliant and during mechanical ventilation air finds its way to areas of least resistance – the upper lung. Further falls in PaO_2 may be caused by a reduction in cardiac output as intrathoracic pressure becomes more positive during mechanical ventilation.

Hypoxaemia is common during thoracic surgery mainly due to:

- Shunting of blood through collapsed upper lung
- Shunting of blood through lower lung because of micro-atelectasis

---

Hypoxic pulmonary vasoconstriction as a compensatory mechanism may have a minor beneficial role during surgery. During one-lung anaesthesia, although alveolar ventilation is reduced, hypercapnia does not usually cause concern as the anaesthetist ensures that the minute volume is maintained at a level appropriate for the two lungs (even though one is collapsed).

In chronic pulmonary disorders the circulation to diseased lungs is often considerably reduced and because some adaptation has therefore occurred prior to surgery falls in PaO_2 may not be as great as in patients presenting for other types of thoracic surgery with normal lungs, e.g. oesophagus.

Sometimes hypoxaemia during surgery demands additional intervention and CPAP (continuous positive airway pressure) to the operative lung and PEEP (positive end expiratory pressure) to the dependent lung may be used.

Following pulmonary resection the anaesthetist confirms with the surgeon whether or not suture lines and lung surfaces have air leaks. This may be determined by, for example, applying positive pressure via the ventilator through the double lumen tube and observing for the presence of gas bubbles in the pleural cavity. If an air leak is excessive then corrective surgery or suturing will be necessary, although a small air leak will diminish as the remaining lung tissue expands. Following lobectomy the anaesthetist ensures that the tracheobronchial tree is clear and the lungs are reinflated manually. Two chest drains are inserted and connected to an underwater seal drain. These drains are left open. Following a pneumonectomy the non-operated lung is reinflated and centralised. It is important that the mediastinum is positioned correctly otherwise serious haemodynamic and pulmonary changes can occur. This is achieved either by leaving in a chest drain which is clamped and later unclamped for a minute every hour or by the surgeon aspirating air from the hemithorax with a syringe.

At the end of the procedure the double lumen tube is changed for a conventional endotracheal tube. Spontaneous ventilation is once more established at the end of surgery, and once extubated, the patient is positioned well-supported with pillows, supplementary oxygen given and the immediate post-operative care given in a high dependency area. It may be necessary for some patients to receive a period of intermittent positive pressure ventilation post-operatively in which case transfer to an intensive care unit will be needed. Fast track for early tracheal extubation is based on sufficient gas exchange with an $SaO_2 > 90$ on FIO_2 of 0.40 and stable cardiovascular conditions. The patient must be awake and orientated with recovery of all protective reflexes.

Video-assisted thoracic surgery (VATS)

Surgeons are continuing to develop video-assisted thoracic surgical techniques for both diagnostic and therapeutic purposes and this has been made possible by the developments in video technology and instrumentation. Preparation of the patient is as for standard thoracotomy, and once intubated with a double lumen tube the patient is similarly positioned laterally with the operated side uppermost. The surgeon makes a small incision which follows the same line as the usual anterolateral incision and any additional entry points are positioned so that some of these can be used for intercostal drainage at the end of surgery. Several ports allow the surgeon to use various instruments according to the procedure being performed. The upper lung is collapsed and once the thoracoscope has been introduced a video camera and light source are attached allowing the surgeon to view the surgical area on a monitor. If necessary the surgeon can easily revert to open thoracotomy.

Video-assisted surgery results in less tissue damage, and although pain may still be severe immediately following surgery, mobilisation and recovery is usually rapid. VATS has been associated with lower levels of pro-inflammatory cytokines (e.g. interleukin-6) and less effect on specific anti-tumour immunity and non-specific secondary immunity (Craig *et al.* 2001). Although post-operative markers of inflammation and impaired immune function are reduced, the clinical significance has yet to be shown (Moffatt *et al.* 2002). Intravenous opioids are usually sufficient but some procedures involving the pleura can still be extremely painful, requiring an epidural. Intercostal drainage is usual for a short period to facilitate inflation of the operated lung post-operatively and persistent air leak may be troublesome. The principles of nursing care following VATS remain the same and although a relatively safe procedure the following complications are possible (Rao *et al.* 1999):

- Subcutaneous emphysema
- Bleeding requiring transfusion
- Cardiac arrhythmias
- Infection
- Dissemination of malignant tumours
- Atelectasis
- Pneumonia
- Empyema
- Wound infection
- Trocar injury
- Myocardial infarction
- Death

Pleurectomy, lung biopsy, drainage of effusions/talc pleurodesis and lung volume reduction surgery have been by VATS. Although VATS may be used for staging in some patients, lung resection remains controversial, as clearance of tumour may be less effective than with open thoracotomy.

Lung volume reduction

In emphysema there is permanent abnormal enlargement of the distal air spaces with destruction of the bronchiole wall. With a loss of elastin due to proteases there is an increase in compliance but decrease in elastic recoil, resulting in air trapping with hyperinflation of the lungs. With flattening of the diaphragm the lungs are at a mechanical disadvantage and the work of breathing is increased, particularly during the expiratory phase, often resulting in collapse of distal airways.

In 1957 (Brantigan *et al.* 1959) it was hypothesised that removal of localised emphysematous areas might provide benefit by:

- Re-expansion of the more normal lung by allowing its elastic recoil properties to exert radial traction on small airways and thus promote their patency during expiration
- An overall decrease in lung volume promoting better chest wall mechanics and restoring a more normal diaphragm configuration.

Several trials have now shown that in patients with emphysema, lung volume reduction can alter lung function, increase walking distance and improve quality of life (Geddes *et al.* 2000; Goodnight-White *et al.* 2001). Surgery is often performed through a median sternotomy reducing morbidity associated with bilateral thoracotomy and 20–30% of the most diseased portions of each lung are removed. One-lung anaesthesia is used with a double lumen tube and the procedure usually involves bilateral surgical removal of lung tissue and staple lines reinforced with bovine pericardium strips (Cooper 1995). Four chest drains are usually inserted and, to avoid injury to lung tissue, suction at a reduced level of − 10 cm of water pressure is applied. Some surgeons may avoid suction completely.

Post-operatively, hypotension may occur due to fluid restriction. In addition, the epidural can result in sympathetic blockade and peripheral vasodilation. Heat loss during the peri-operative period may result in hypothermia and prolonged bleeding times so steps should be taken to restore normal body temperature. Haemodynamic status may be further compromised by the development of arrhythmias during the first few days following surgery.

Because of the long history of emphysema there can be significant pulmonary problems in the immediate post-operative period following lung volume reduction. As with all patients following thoracic surgery, therapeutic interventions are employed to minimise the risk of atelectasis, pneumonia and respiratory failure.

Although early use of lung volume reduction often involved patients with severe end stage emphysema, preliminary findings from the National Emphysema Treatment Trial (NETT 2001) have warned against performing surgery on patients with a low forced expiratory volume in 1 second (<20% predicted) or very low transfer factor (<20% predicted), because of a high risk of death. As a result, many patients are now excluded from surgery. However, an alternative procedure for volume reduction using a bronchoscopic approach (Ingenito *et al.* 2001) shows promise, but as yet there have been no trials in humans and many questions remain (Toma *et al.* 2002).

References

Abrahamov, D., Bhatnagar, G. & Goldma, B. (2000) When is surgery indicated? In: Soltoski, P., Karamanoukian, H. & Slaerno, T. (eds) *Cardiac Surgery Secrets*. Hanley & Belfus, Philadelphia.

Arcasoy, S.M. & Kotloff, R.M. (1999) Medical progress: lung transplantation. *New England Journal of Medicine* **340**: 1081.

Barr, J. & Donner, A. (1995) Optimal intravenous dosing strategies for sedatives and analgesics in the intensive care unit. *Critical Care Clinics* **11**: 827.

Bloomfield, P. (2002) Choice of heart valve prosthesis. *Heart* **87**: 583–9.

Bradshaw, P., Jamrozik, K., Le, M., Gilfillan, I. & Thompson, C. (2002) Mortality and recurrent cardiac events after coronary artery bypass graft: long term outcomes in a population study. *Heart* **88**(5): 488–94.

Brantigan, O.C., Mueller, E. & Kress, M.B. (1959) A surgical approach to pulmonary emphysema. *American Review of Respiratory Diseases* **80**: 194–206.

Cooper, J.D. (1995) Technique to reduce air leaks after resection of emphysematous lung. *Annals of Thoracic Surgery* **57**: 1038–9.

Craig, S.R., Leaver, H.A., Yap, P.L. *et al.* (2001) Acute phase response following minimal access and conventional thoracic surgery. *European Journal of Cardiothoracic Surgery* **20**: 455–63.

De Amicis, V., Ascione, R., Ianelli, G., Di Tommaso, L., Monaco, M. & Spampinato, N. (1997) Aortic valve replacement through a minimally invasive approach. *Texas Heart Institute* **14**(4): 353–5.

De Jaegere, P. & Suyker, W. (2002) Off-pump coronary artery bypass surgery. *Heart* **88**(3): 313–18.

Edgerton, J.R. & Michelson, L. (2000) *Beating Heart Surgery: Moving from Revolutionary to Routine*. Medtronic, USA.

Geddes, D., Davies, M., Koyama, H. *et al.* (2000) Effect of lung volume reduction surgery in patients with severe emphysema. *New England Journal of Medicine* **343**: 239–45.

Goodnight-White, S., Jones, J.W., Baaklini, W.A. *et al.* (2001) Lung volume reduction surgery (LVRS) in patients with severe emphysema: 1 year follow up. *American Journal of Respiratory Critical Care Medicine* **163**: A486.

Ghosh, S. & Latimer, R.D. (1999) *Thoracic Anaesthesia. Principles and Practice.* Butterworth-Heinemann, Oxford.

Gothard, J.W.W. (1993) *Anaesthesia for Thoracic Surgery.* Blackwell Science, London.

Hayden, A. (1998) Transmyocardial revascularisation. *Registered Nurse* **61**(5): 44–8.

Hazelrigg, S.R., Landreneau, R.J., Boley, T.M., *et al.* (1991) The effect of muscle sparing versus standard posterolateral thoracotomy on pulmonary function, muscle strength and postoperative pain. *Journal of Thoracic and Cardiovascular Surgery* **101**: 394.

Ibrahim, M., Venn, G., Young, C. & Chambers, D. (1999) A clinical comparative study between crystalloid and blood-based St Thomas' hospital cardioplegic solution. *European Journal of Cardiothoracic Surgery* **15**(1): 75–83.

Ingenito, E.P., Reilly, J.J., Mentzer, S.J. *et al.* (2001) Bronchoscopic volume reduction. A safe and effective alternative to surgical therapy for emphysema. *American Journal of Respiratory Critical Care Medicine* **164**: 295–301.

Jansen, E., Borts, C., Lahpor, J. *et al.* (1998) Coronary artery bypass grafting without cardiopulmonary bypass using the octopus method: results of the first one hundred patients. *Journal of Thoracic and Cardiovascular Surgery* **116**(1): 60–67.

Jarpe, M. (1992) Nursing care of patients receiving long term infusion of neuromuscular blocking agents. *Critical Care Nurse* **12**(7): 58–63.

Julian, D.G. (1989) *Diseases of the Heart.* Elsevier Science, London.

Keffelmann, T., Schwarz, E., Skobel, C., Petek, O. & Hanrath, P. (2000) Ischaemic pre-conditioning: does this animal experiment phenomenon have clinical relevance? *Clinical Medicine* **95**(10): 559–68.

Khan, I. & Nair, C. (2002) Clinical, diagnostic and management perspectives of aortic dissection. *Chest* **122**(1): 311–28.

Kolker, A.C. (1997) Selection of anaesthetic agents for thoracotomy. *Chest Surgery Clinics of North America* **7**(4): 707–19.

Lichtenberg, A., Hagl, C., Harringer, W., Klima, U. & Haverich, A. (2000) Effects of minimal invasive coronary artery bypass on pulmonary function and postoperative pain. *Annals of Thoracic Surgery* **70**(2): 461–5.

Mathews, R. (2002) Surgical procedures and nursing care for coronary heart disease. *Professional Nurse* **17**(5): 304–7.

Moffatt, S.D., Mitchell, J.D. & Whyte, R.I. (2002) Role of video-assisted thoracoscopic surgery and classic thoracotomy in lung cancer management. *Current Opinion in Pulmonary Medicine* **8**(4): 281–6.

NETT (National Emphysema Treatment Trial Research Group) (2001) Patients at high risk of death after lung volume reduction surgery. *New England Journal of Medicine* **345**: 1075–83.

Ng, P., Chua, A., Swanson, M., Koutlas, T., Chitwood, W. & Elbery, J. (2000) Anterior thoracotomy wound complications in minimally invasive direct coronary artery bypass. *Annals of Thoracic Surgery* **69**(5): 1338–40.

Pillai, R. & Wright, J. (1999) Technical aspects of coronary artery surgery. In: Pillai, R. & Wright, J. (eds) *Surgery for Ischemic Heart Disease.* Oxford University Press, Oxford.

Plummer, S., Hartley, M. & Vaughn, R.S. (1998) Anaesthesia for telescopic procedures in the thorax. *British Journal of Anaesthesia* **80**: 223–34.

Rao, A., Bansal, A., Rangraj, M. *et al.* (1999) Video-assisted thoracic surgery (VATS). *Heart and Lung: The Journal of Acute and Critical Care* **28**(1): 15–19.

Seijo, L.M. & Sterman, D.H. (2001) Medical progress. *Interventional Pulmonology* **344**(10): 740–49.

Strandberg, A., Tokics, L., Brismar., B. *et al.* (1986) Atelectasis during anaesthesia and in the postoperative period. *Acta Anaesthesiologica Scandinavica* **30**: 154.

Strollo, D.C., Rosado de Christensen, M.L. & Jett, J.R. (1997) Primary mediastinal tumours: Part 1. Tumours of the anterior mediastinum. *Chest* **112**: 511.

Taggart, D. (2002) Bilateral internal mammary artery grafting: are BIMA better? *Heart* **88**: 7–9.

Toma, T.P., Goldstraw, P. & Geddes, D.M. (2002) Lung volume reduction surgery. *Thorax* **57**(1): 5.

Wang, C. & Pinsky, D. (2000) Contribution of inflammation to reperfusion injury. *Journal of Cardiac Surgery* **15**: 149–62.

6

Post-operative Care following Cardiothoracic Surgery

All patients following cardiothoracic surgery will have varying degrees of hae-modynamic instability and pulmonary impairment with hypoxaemia. Acute changes of preload, pulmonary dynamics, autonomic nervous tone and blood properties will tax the already compromised physiological systems. The heart will also be placed under considerable stress and this may lead to post-operative morbidity, even in patients with previously healthy hearts. This chapter considers some of the issues in the care and management of the patient following cardio-thoracic surgery.

The maintenance of homeostasis in the post-operative period is crucial and the ability of the heart to raise cardiac output, and for the pulmonary system to maximise gaseous exchange is necessary for a successful post-operative period. Continuation of the stress response in the immediate post-operative period may be maladaptive and a major contributing factor in the development of many of the post-operative complications. Along with other members of the team, the nurse has a key role in helping to modify the stress response by employing effective strategies in the pre- and post-operative periods. This is particularly important regarding assessment, sedation and pain relief and in the creation of a safe care environment that is conducive to maximising the healing process.

Prevention, early identification and correction of tissue hypoxia are important skills in caring for the critically ill patient and require an understanding of oxygen transport, delivery and consumption (Leach & Treacher 2002). The development of metabolic acidosis, accumulation of lactate (>2 mmol/l), a fall in mixed venous oxygen saturation together with oliguria and impaired consciousness are indi-cative of worsening oxygen delivery. Although raising FIO_2 may improve the PaO_2, additional parameters reflecting the effectiveness of DO_2 must be moni-tored. The oxygen-carrying capacity of the blood must be increased, but increasing the haemoglobin concentration too much may result in increased viscosity with impaired flow through the microcirculation, and levels around 10 g/dl are considered acceptable (Hebert *et al.* 1999). An effective cardiac output is necessary to transport the oxygenated blood to the tissues, and left ventricular function therefore is an important consideration. Shivering, pyrexia, pain, anxiety and sympathomimetic agents may all increase oxygen consumption further in the early post-operative period and mechanical ventilation, sedation, analgesia and, if necessary, therapeutic paralysis will reduce VO_2 (Leach & Treacher 2002).

Pulmonary changes following cardiothoracic surgery

When vital capacity and functional residual capacity are reduced during surgery they are unlikely to return to normal until well into the post-operative period. This together with the inevitable compression of lung tissue and poor diaphragmatic movement will lead to micro-atelectasis, a common event following cardio-thoracic surgery. If loss of lung volume is significant this will be detectable on chest radiography. Atelectasis will cause ventilation perfusion mismatch with a right to left shunt, causing reduced PaO_2 and oxygen saturations. Accumulating secretions in the airways during general anaesthesia will also contribute to atelectasis and may lead to post-operative pneumonia.

A number of additional intra-operative factors may contribute towards the development of pulmonary problems and these are outlined in Fig. 6.1.

In cardiac surgery it is the utilisation of cardiopulmonary bypass (CPB) that is responsible for pulmonary changes such as a decrease in functional residual capacity (FRC) (Taggart *et al.* 1993; Kochamba *et al.* 2000), increased lung permeability and reduced surfactant (Royston *et al.* 1985; Haslam *et al.* 1997). During thoracic surgery the lung on the operated side is often collapsed resulting in a right to left shunt. Cardiac and thoracic surgical procedures usually require median sternotomy and posterolateral incisions, respectively, and these incisions alone affect the integrity of the chest wall, reducing compliance. With compression atelectasis and decreased compliance the work of breathing is increased significantly. As a result, patients often show decreased tidal volumes and increased respiratory rates, and while this will maintain minute volume in the short term, high respiratory rates will increase oxygen consumption and lead to muscle fatigue. If the patient is unduly distressed because of increased respiratory effort then this should be investigated and corrected. Worsening hypoxaemia, tachycardia, tachypnoea, fever and increased anxiety may all be indicative of atelectasis or some other developing respiratory problem. Figure 6.2 shows the changes which occur with post-operative atelectasis.

A significant number of patients requiring surgery today are elderly, and age-related changes in the respiratory system and a history of smoking may contribute to pulmonary complications (Kheradmand *et al.* 1997). In the elderly, for example, there is a gradual breakdown of elastin and cross-linking of collagen that impairs lung elastic recoil, a decline in respiratory muscle strength and endurance with less thoracic cage compliance. With increasing age, closing capacity is nearer functional residual capacity which results in airway collapse during normal breathing. Positioning during and immediately following surgery may exaggerate this effect.

Changes in gas exchange as a result of surgery can continue well into the post-operative period and the nurse must be alert for signs of deteriorating pulmonary status. Most patients will receive supplementary oxygen, and with PaO_2 values possibly underestimating any ventilation abnormality, additional signs of pulmonary compromise must be watched for.

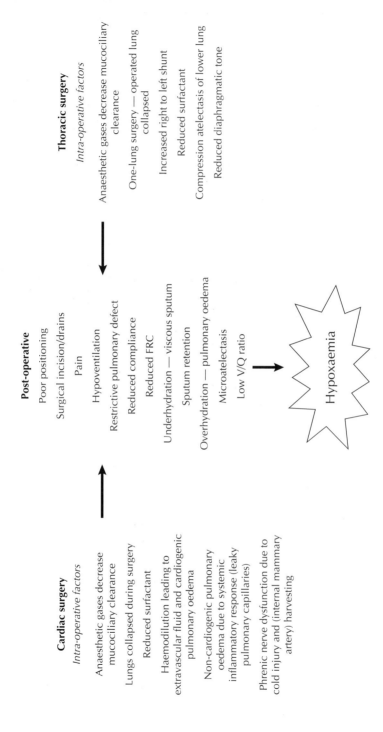

Cardiac surgery

Intra-operative factors

Anaesthetic gases decrease mucociliary clearance

Lungs collapsed during surgery

Reduced surfactant

Haemodilution leading to extravascular fluid and cardiogenic pulmonary oedema

Non-cardiogenic pulmonary oedema due to systemic inflammatory response (leaky pulmonary capillaries)

Phrenic nerve dysfunction due to cold injury and (internal mammary artery) harvesting

Post-operative

Poor positioning

Surgical incision/drains

Pain

Hypoventilation

Restrictive pulmonary defect

Reduced compliance

Reduced FRC

Underhydration — viscous sputum

Sputum retention

Overhydration — pulmonary oedema

Microatelectasis

Low V/Q ratio

Thoracic surgery

Intra-operative factors

Anaesthetic gases decrease mucociliary clearance

One-lung surgery — operated lung collapsed

Increased right to left shunt

Reduced surfactant

Compression atelectasis of lower lung

Reduced diaphragmatic tone

Hypoxaemia

Fig. 6.1   Pulmonary effects of cardiac and thoracic surgery.

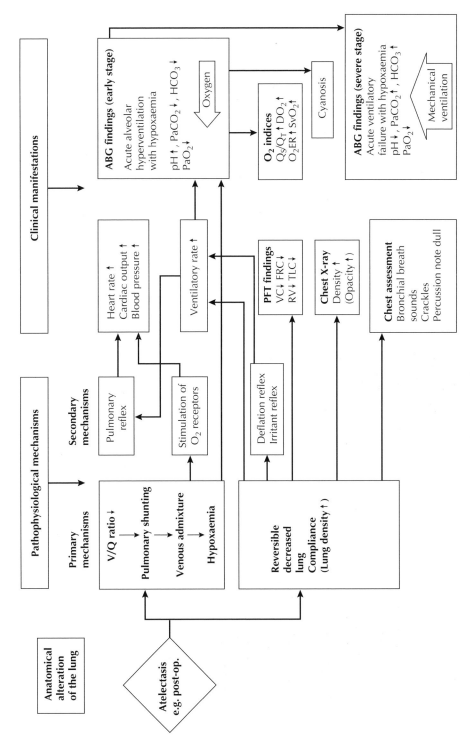

Fig. 6.2 Hypoxaemia as a result of atelectasis. From Des Jardins *et al.* (1997), with permission.

The following sections consider issues specifically related to cardiac and thoracic surgery before exploring additional aspects of care in the post-operative period. A comprehensive table setting out issues in the post-operative management of the patient following cardiac surgery is presented as an appendix to this chapter.

Specific care issues following cardiac surgery

Historically, the person who has undergone cardiac surgery has been cared for in the intensive care setting. More recently, however, the fast-track principle, although originally designed to eliminate long waiting lists (Ranganathan 1989), has changed the emphasis of care from one that is 'high tech to high touch' (Riley 1995). Utilising the principles discussed in Chapter 4, careful selection is made of those patients most likely to benefit from fast-tracking. Table 6.1 suggests guidelines for identifying such patients.

Table 6.1   Fast-track criteria

- Age <70 years
- Left ventricular ejection >30%
- Left ventricular ejection >50% if myocardial infarction within previous month
- Respiratory parameters within normal limits
- Renal function within normal limits
- Liver function within normal limits
- Coagulation within normal limits
- No recent alcohol or recreational drug abuse
- Systemic hypertension controlled pre-operatively
- No previous cerebrovascular accident
- Planned surgery
- First operation for revascularisation
- No insulin-dependent diabetes
- Body weight <20% over ideal weight

Pulmonary issues

Intra-operative care should facilitate early extubation, which should occur either prior to leaving the operating room or soon after the return to the recovery unit. For this reason the pharmacological reversal of any residual effects of muscle relaxants or anaesthetic agents is needed and the patient should be completely rewarmed before leaving the operating room. Sedation may reduce the stress response often associated with adverse outcome; however, prolonged use increases the need for mechanical ventilation and a period in the intensive care unit (ICU). This is in opposition to current practices of early extubation and fast-tracking (Doering 1997; Dunstan & Riddle 1997). The use of a short-acting sedative drug such as propofol, combined with analgesia, will decrease the stress response and has been shown to reduce myocardial ischaemia (Hall *et al.* 1997). It may therefore be useful in the immediate post-operative period. This will allow the patient to verbalise their anxieties or need for pain relief while still allowing for early extubation. Analgesia through the intermittent use of intravenous opiates or patient-controlled analgesia is effective to reduce pain and facilitate deep breathing and early mobilisation.

Where early extubation is not an option, the patient is transferred to the ICU and volume cycled mechanical ventilation is established, usually with a synchronised intermittent mandatory ventilatory mode. If arterial blood gases are acceptable then FIO_2 is maintained at 0.40. The patient remains sedated and mechanically ventilated thereby reducing the work of breathing. Continuous post-operative sedation and analgesia may reduce the incidence or severity of any post-operative myocardial ischaemic episodes and thus contributes towards fewer adverse events (Reyes *et al.* 1997).

Weaning from mechanical ventilation is usually quite rapid and follows a short trial period of spontaneous breathing via the endotracheal tube and T piece or CPAP. Pulmonary and haemodynamic parameters are monitored carefully during this time to see if extubation is possible (see Table 6.2). Delayed weaning from mechanical ventilation in patients following cardiac surgery may be due to (Gothard & Kelleher 1999):

- Pre-existing pulmonary disease
- Left ventricular failure
- Pneumonia
- Neurological damage
- Pneumothorax or pleural effusion
- Phrenic nerve injury associated with the use of topical slush
- Acute lung injury associated with CPB including acute respiratory distress syndrome (ARDS)

Table 6.2 Parameters for weaning from mechanical ventilation

- Alert and able to follow verbal commands
- Haemodynamic stability (MAP >80 mmHg without large doses of vasodilators or inotropes other than dopamine (<5 mcg/kg/min); no untreated arrhythmias
- Minimal chest tube drainage (<50 ml/h)
- Normothermia (>35.5°C)
- Arterial blood gases: PaO_2 >10 kPa
  PCO_2 <5.5 kPa
  pH 7.32–7.45
- Respiratory rate <24/min
- Ventilatory support no more than 50% O_2 and PEEP <5 cm H_2O

Extra vigilance should be exercised where the internal mammary artery has been used for coronary artery revascularisation and the pleural cavity has been opened. This can increase the risk of pulmonary problems (Gilbert *et al.* 1996).

Mild pulmonary complications are to be expected and these may include chest infections caused by limited mobility, pain, inadequate pain relief and shallow breathing with the sternal wound site. The pre-operative condition of the patient also plays a significant part in the development of such complications. Age, obesity, massive blood transfusions, low cardiac output and sepsis have all been implicated. Yet a more recent study also indicated a clear correlation between pulmonary complications and other factors such as hypoalbuminaemia, emergency surgery, pre-operative raised pulmonary artery pressures and a history of CVA (Rady *et al.* 1997). The use of the pre-operative period to identify those at increased risk of pulmonary complications, and to start pre-operative interventions, is clear. Atelectasis may develop secondary to hypoventilation and will be compounded by the reduced production of surfactant that occurs when the lungs are left deflated for a period of time, as during CPB. Less commonly, adult respiratory distress syndrome develops. This is largely thought to occur secondary to increased capillary permeability following CPB. When it does occur, it is associated with increased mortality.

Haemodynamic status

Low cardiac output can be a serious complication following cardiac surgery. In patients with pre-existing left ventricular dysfunction, low cardiac output in the post-operative period is not surprising, yet may return to normal over the following days or weeks. When the depressed left ventricular function occurs at rest it is likely to be ischaemic in origin and the term 'hibernating myocardium' is used. This indicates that the myocardial cells remain viable but contraction is chronically depressed. Hence, once the blood supply to the myocardium is restored, left ventricular function may improve. It must be recognised, however, that as poor left ventricular function is not always due to a hibernating myocardium, function may not improve with cardiac surgery. Patients that have developed heart failure should not be assured that their heart function will necessarily improve, although their symptoms should reduce.

For others, post-operative left ventricular dysfunction is not anticipated from the pre-operative assessment, and the term 'stunned myocardium' may be a more appropriate term, necessitating a short period of post-operative inotropic support. During cardiac surgery, despite good myocardial protection outlined in the previous chapter, the myocardial cells may experience brief periods of ischaemia. This may lead to post-ischaemic contraction dysfunction, lasting for several hours or even weeks. Indeed, Kloner *et al.* (2001) suggest that this transient depression of the left ventricular function may be fairly common despite the increasing attention given to myocardial protection. This raises the importance of improving myocardial protection and ischaemic preconditioning and indicates another potential advantage of beating heart surgery. The two major hypotheses for myocardial stunning include the effect of oxygen free radicals on reperfusion (Bojar 1999) and a loss of sensitivity of the myofilaments to calcium alongside reduced calcium storage (Elasser *et al.* 1997). It is likely that these two hypotheses are not mutually exclusive and that a combination of the two is responsible for the changes observed.

When poor ventricular function is anticipated, invasive monitoring should be used in the immediate post-operative period. It is likely that a pulmonary flotation catheter or left atrial line will have been inserted intra-operatively and should be used to guide the post-operative management. An intensive care bed should be organised. Treatment of low cardiac output in these situations requires the careful manipulation of haemodynamic parameters, administration of inotropic agents and the optimisation of filling pressures as illustrated in the first case study below. In rare instances, an intra-aortic balloon pump or left ventricular assist device may be necessary to maintain cardiac output while the heart recovers from the immediate insult. When low cardiac output occurs during the course of an otherwise normal post-operative period, alternative causes should be detected, such as electrolyte abnormalities, arrhythmias, cardiac tamponade, bleeding or sudden vasodilation. This is illustrated by the second case study.

Case study 1: Low cardiac output

Mr Jones, a 54-year-old gentleman, has undergone coronary artery bypass grafting and returned from the theatre approximately 3 hours ago. Since then he has warmed up slowly and now has a central temperature of 35°C. He is cool peripherally to touch with poor capillary refill.

Additional data records the following values:

Heart rate | 110 bpm (sinus tachycardia)
Blood pressure | 95/50 mmHg
RAP | 14 mmHg
ABGs: PaO_2 | 11.0 kPa
$PaCO_2$ | 5.2 kPa
HCO_3 | 23 mmol/l
BE | 4.5
O_2 saturation | 96% on 50% O_2 on IPPV
K^+ | 4.5 mmol/l
Urine output after initial diuresis has tailed off to 20 ml/h (weight = 80 kg)
Chest drainage | 50 ml/h
Haemoglobin | 10.0 g/dl

Mr Jones is demonstrating all the signs of a reduced cardiac output; both his central and peripheral temperatures remain low and his feet feel cold to touch. His urine output and blood pressure are low. The heart rate at 110 bpm demonstrates the normal compensatory mechanism to the low cardiac output.

The right atrial pressure (RAP) is high and the haemoglobin level is within normal limits. This is not consistent with hypovolaemia as a cause for the reduced cardiac output. The probable cause is decreased myocardial contractility due to myocardial ischaemia, infarction or stunning.

Treatment

A 12 lead ECG was recorded for signs of ischaemia or infarction and a low dose of intravenous nitrate therapy was started. This would eliminate any coronary artery spasm and increase the myocardial oxygen supply while reducing myocardial oxygen demand.

At this stage the low urine output should not be treated with a fluid challenge as the RAP is high. Instead, a low-dose intravenous infusion of dopamine could be started to improve renal perfusion and the inotropic action of the heart. Alternatively, dobutamine could be used for its inotropic effect while having a lesser effect upon the heart rate.

Mr Jones should be kept sedated and ventilated until his cardiac output shows signs of responding to the treatment. If Mr Jones' cardiac function remains poor, additional inotropic drugs may be considered or the intra-aortic balloon pump.

Conclusion

Mr Jones was developing cardiogenic shock. Myocardial contraction should be helped through increasing myocardial oxygen supply through good oxygenation and nitrate therapy. Myocardial oxygen consumption should be minimised through reducing the work of breathing. Myocardial contraction can be enhanced through reducing both the cardiac afterload and preload while an intravenous inotrope will increase myocardial function.

Case study 2: Cardiac tamponade

Mr Smith, a 54-year-old gentleman, has undergone coronary artery bypass grafting and returned from the theatre approximately three hours ago. Since then he has warmed up slowly and now has a central temperature of 35°C. He is cool peripherally to touch with poor capillary refill.

Additional data records the following values:

Heart rate	110 bpm (sinus tachycardia)
Blood pressure	85/50 mmHg
RAP	14 mmHg
ABGs: PaO_2	13.0 kPa
$PaCO_2$	5.2 kPa
HCO_3	23 mmol/l
BE	4.5
O_2 saturation	96% on 50% O_2 on IPPV
K^+	4.5 mmol/l
Urine output after initial diuresis has tailed off to 40 ml/h (weight = 80 kg)	
Chest drainage	<25 ml/h
Haemoglobin	<8.5 g/dl

Note the similarities to the previous case study. Mr Smith is demonstrating all the signs of a reduced cardiac output: both his central and peripheral temperatures remain low and his feet feel cold to touch. His urine output is low, although still above 0.5 ml/kg/h, and his blood pressure is low. The heart rate at 110 bpm demonstrates the normal compensatory mechanism to the low cardiac output. However, the RAP is high while the chest drains have minimal drainage. One possible cause of this low cardiac output therefore is cardiac tamponade, when blood collects around the heart. As the haemoglobin is low, Mr Smith may indeed be bleeding.

Treatment

Mr Smith was sat up to a 45 degree angle to facilitate drainage and release the developing cardiac tamponade. One unit of blood was given to raise the haemoglobin and haematocrit. Raising the haematocrit should also help to improve the blood pressure and the metabolic acidosis should improve slowly as the cardiac output improves and his body temperature rises.

As Mr Smith's condition started to improve a low-dose nitrate was started to assist his rewarming.

Conclusion

Mr Smith was developing a cardiac tamponade, which, if left untreated, would lead to serious haemodynamic compromise and possible cardiac arrest. The high RAP and low blood pressure are classic signs of cardiac tamponade. Consequent to this, the cardiac output will fall and is demonstrated here by the cool temperatures and low blood pressure. The heart rate increases as a compensatory mechanism and the process of cardiogenic shock is beginning. The metabolic acidosis is caused by the low cardiac output. This is compounding the situation by reducing myocardial contractility still further. This cycle should be halted.

This is distinguished from hypovolaemic shock by the right atrial pressure recordings. In Mr Smith's case the RAP was high because the heart was constricted, whereas in the presence of hypovolaemia the RAP reading would be low. The minimal chest tube drainage does not rule out hypovolaemia: it cannot be assumed that there will always be a large blood loss recorded from the chest drains when a patient is hypovolaemic.

Myocardial ischaemia

Myocardial ischaemia can develop in the intra/post-operative period, however, in about 5% of patients undergoing cardiac surgery, the heart is exposed to such severe ischaemia that a myocardial infarction (MI) occurs (Bojar 1999). Causes for this include:

- Severe acidosis
- Long operative procedure
- Long time on CPB

- Lack of collateral blood supply
- Coronary artery spasm
- Inadequate myocardial protection
- Cardiomegaly

Although troponin I is now widely used as a marker of MI, as with creatinine kinase MB (CK-MB) isoenzyme, levels are raised following cardiac surgery and cannot therefore be used to confirm MI. This raises the importance of observing other indicators of myocardial infarction such as the development of new pathological Q waves on the 12 lead ECG or poor R wave progression.

The management of these patients should include strategies to reduce myocardial oxygen imbalance through maximising oxygen supply while reducing demand. Patients who demonstrate myocardial ischaemia should not be extubated early as the increased work of breathing may exacerbate the supply/demand imbalance. Instead, a more prolonged period of sedation and ventilation is appropriate ensuring good oxygenation while increasing myocardial oxygen supply still further through the use of various pharmacological agents (see Table 6.3). The management of various haemodynamic problems is outlined in Table 6.4.

Coronary artery spasm

Coronary artery spasm may occur during the early post-operative period and is recognised by severe haemodynamic collapse, which may lead to cardiac arrest. The cause is unclear although excessive infusions of calcium, hypothermia and increased adrenergic tone have been implicated. The early signs of coronary artery spasm include acute hypotension, ST segment elevation and ventricular arrhythmias. The spasm may be relieved by the intravenous infusion of nitroglycerine, although calcium channel blockers are usually required for severe, acute coronary artery spasm. However, a low dose of nitroglycerine, infused during the first 12 hours following cardiac surgery, may prove effective in eliminating this potentially fatal condition.

Bleeding

Bleeding after cardiac surgery is clearly a risk when considering the number of suture lines, intra-operative heparinisation and platelet depletion or dysfunction associated with CPB. It is standard practice for chest drains to be inserted into the mediastinal area, pericardial region and the pleural space to assist blood drainage and this should be monitored at regular intervals. A gentle suction pressure of around 5 kPa should be applied to the drains. This should maintain a slow, consistent bubbling to the water that creates the underwater seal (Bare El *et al.* 2001). Suction or manipulation of the chest drains that may cause an excessive negative pressure should be avoided. Although there is no strong evidence to suggest how chest drains should be manipulated to encourage drainage and prevent clot formation, the practice of 'milking and stripping' of chest drains is largely avoided in current practice. If blood is thought to be collecting in the mediastinum, drainage through the chest drains may be encouraged through gentle movement of the patient and sitting them up to a 45 degree angle if they are haemodynamically stable. Bleeding can lead to serious haemodynamic consequences associated with hypovolaemic shock. If excessive bleeding is recognised it is important to eliminate the cause.

Cardiac tamponade

Cardiac tamponade may occur when blood or fluid collects in the pericardial space. The pericardial sac is fibrous with little elasticity. A gentle stretching of the pericardium may accommodate a slow accumulation of fluid. In contrast, the rapid accumulation of fluid will compress the heart, preventing diastolic filling and reducing cardiac output. An acute cardiac tamponade, therefore, may develop when excessive bleeding results in clots forming within drainage tubes, preventing further drainage so that blood collects within the pericardial cavity. Coagulopathies associated with CPB, combined with inadequate surgical haemostasis, are more common causes of excessive bleeding, although excessive strain on suture lines caused by inadequately controlled high blood pressure has also been cited. Early tamponade may also occur when intracardiac monitoring catheters are removed, such as a left atrial line, or following the removal of epicardial pacing wires. The classic symptoms of a cardiac tamponade are known as Beck's triad: the heart is small and the heart sounds are muffled, the venous pressure is elevated and the systemic arterial pressure is decreased. The clinical signs are outlined in Table 6.5.

When cardiac tamponade is suspected, non-invasive echocardiography may be useful. Cardiac tamponade may be a very late complication occurring up to 6 months after surgery (Johnston & McKinley 2000).

An emergency exploratory sternotomy, either in the operating room or at the bedside, is a lifesaving procedure that may be necessary to treat major haemorrhage, acute hypotension, cardiac tamponade or cardiac arrest. Possibly as many as 3% of patients require re-exploration for excessive bleeding (Slaughter *et al.* 2001). Clearly, the nurse plays an important part in recognising the warning signs of a deteriorating condition. Although the atrial suture lines are common sites for bleeding, discrete sites may not be discovered on re-exploration of the operative sites. This highlights the necessity to treat any coagulopathies first, before exploration of the mediastinum and a repeat anaesthetic to the patient who is already haemodynamically compromised.

Arrhythmias

Arrhythmias following cardiac surgery occur commonly and for a variety of reasons. The increased secretion of catecholamines resulting from the stress response shifts potassium into the cell and may lead to hypokalaemia. The hypokalaemic cell is more negatively charged and requires a greater trigger for depolarisation. Meanwhile, the ventricular cells are able to spontaneously depolarise and ventricular arrhythmias, such as premature ventricular contractions (PVCs), may result. Conversely, the hyperkalaemic cell becomes partially

Table 6.3 Examples of pharmacological agents used post-operatively

Drug	Action	Indications	Side-effects	Nursing implications
Dopamine endogenous catecholamine-precursor of norepinephrine	Inotropic with some chronotropic effects Haemodynamic effects are dose dependent Dopaminergic receptors stimulated at low doses result in increase urinary output and increased sodium excretion (1.0–2.0 mcg/kg/min) β-1 increase myocardial contractility and α-1 vasoconstriction of smooth muscle, renal and mesenteric vascular beds at moderate doses (2.0–10 mcg/kg/min) Alpha properties dominate at high doses causing potent vasoconstriction of arteries and veins (10 mcg/kg/min). Can be combined with vasodilator to counter α activity	Increase contractility in congestive heart failure Increase blood pressure in hypotensive or shocked states Administration of low-dose dopamine to critically ill patients at risk of renal failure does not offer clinical significant protection from renal dysfunction	Pulmonary congestion due to increase preload Pulmonary oedema if left ventricular function is poor Tachycardia and dysrhythmias particularly in volume-depleted patients Headaches Ischaemia due to increased MVO_2 Nausea and vomiting	Administration via an infusion pump Administer through central or peripheral line. Central line administration for concentrations over 2 mg/ml Continuous cardiac and arterial pressure monitoring Correct hypovolaemic states Observe for extravasation and subcutaneous necrosis around infusion site Incompatible with many alkaline solutions Wean off gradually
Dobutamine synthetic catecholamine	Inotropic with minimal chronotropic effect Stimulate β-1 receptors at lower doses and β-1 and β-2 at higher doses (7.5 mcg/kg/min). Minimal α-1 (vasoconstriction) antagonised by β-2 effects Increased myocardial contractility and vasodilation at higher doses decreasing afterload and SVR Increases cardiac output/stroke volume therefore MVO_2 Preload and afterload reduction through vasodilation	Congestive cardiac failure and other states of decreased cardiac output Pulmonary congestion Initial dose 2.5–5 mcg/kg/min Usual 2.5–10 mcg/kg/min Maximum 40 mcg/kg/min *Contra-indications:* idiopathic hypertrophic subaortic stenosis	Ventricular ectopics, ischaemia and chest pain due to increased MVO_2 Nausea and vomiting Down-regulation of receptors which can be overcome with intermittent dosing	Administration via an infusion pump Drug concentrations above 5 mg in 1 ml must be given via a central line Continuous cardiac and haemodynamic monitoring Titrate in accordance with prescribed haemodynamic parameters Correct hypovolaemic states, if urine output increases monitor potassium and magnesium levels Many drug incompatibilities Wean off gradually

	Action	Indications/Doses	Side effects	Nursing
Phosphodiesterase-III inhibitors or 'inodilators'	Inotropic – inhibition of phosphodiesterase, raises level of Camp Vasodilator – phosphodiesterase inhibitors exert a direct relaxed effect on vascular smooth muscle resulting in vasodilation of venous and arterial vasculature reducing preload and afterload	Falling cardiac output and when other inotropes cause tachycardia Poor right ventricular contraction and pulmonary hypertension Amrinone 10–15 mcg/kg/min Milrinone 0.375–0.75 mcg/kg/min	**Amrinone** Thrombocytopenia Cardiac arrhythmias Nausea Vomiting Hepatic function abnormalities	Continuous infusion via an infusion pump Continuous cardiac and arterial pressure monitoring Correct hypovolaemic states Thrombocytopenia reported with amrinone (platelet count important), rarely with milrinone Long half-life, having haemodynamic effects for several hours – continue to monitor as effects start to wear off Wean gradually
Amrinone	Systemic vasodilator effect (70%), increasing myocardial contraction, cardiac output and stroke volume through phosphodiesterase inhibition and increased Ca^{++} transport across cell membrane raising level of intracellular Ca^{++}. Inotropic effect accounts for 30% of its action		**Milrinone** Angina Flushing Headaches Hyperthyroidism Arrhythmias	
Milrinone	Potent inotrope and vasodilatory effects reducing SVR, improving cardiac output, coronary perfusion and myocardial relaxation with only 5% rise in MVO_2			

Contd

Table 6.3 *Contd*

Drug	Action	Indications	Side-effects	Nursing implications
Epinephrine endogenous catecholamine synthesised from tyrosine in the adrenal medulla	β-1 effects at low doses increase myocardial contractility β-2 effects – vasodilation and bronchodilation α-1 vasoconstriction β-centrally inhibits norepinephrine when epinephrine at high doses Increases glucagon by increasing glycogenolysis and decreases insulin production (β₂) Major effect: increases blood pressure, systemic vascular resistance, automaticity of the heart, coronary and cerebral blood flow *Contra-indications*: hyperthyroidism	Cardiac arrest Epinephrine increases susceptibility of ventricular fibrillation to defibrillation, used as first line drug for ventricular fibrillation First line drug for pulseless electrical activity (PEA) 1 mg (10 ml of 1:10 000) Poor cardiac output (low dose) Anaphylaxis	Increase myocardial contractility at expense of increased MVO₂ which may increase angina or pain Severe hypertension Hyperglycaemia Central nervous system excitability – anxiety, headache, dizziness Mydriasis at high doses Can cause metabolic acidosis	Administration via an infusion pump Administered via central line Must not be administered or added to alkaline solutions (e.g. sodium bicarbonate) Continuous cardiac monitoring – observe for tachycardia and arrhythmias Arterial pressure monitoring Increased α activity at high doses increasing vasoconstriction and blood pressure therefore monitor for extravasation around infusion site Titrate in accordance with prescribed haemodynamic parameters Blood glucose and potassium levels Wean slowly
Norepinephrine an endogenous catecholamine	α-1 properties dominate, potent vasoconstriction and increased afterload raising systemic blood pressure Increases afterload and contractility with an increase in MVO₂, heart rate remains constant Reduces local tissue perfusion	Especially useful in hypotensive states with low systemic vascular resistance such as sepsis Starting dose (especially following cardiac surgery as patients warm and vasodilate: 2–100 mcg/min *Interactions*: Tricyclic antidepressants and MAO inhibitors increase norepinephrine effects	Increasing afterload and contractility with an increase in MVO₂ resulting in a decrease in cardiac output Peripheral hypoperfusion causing renal, abdominal visceral and skeletal muscle ischaemia	Administration via an infusion pump Administered via central line Continuous cardiac monitoring for increasing angina, ventricular ectopic (myocardial stress) Arterial pressure monitoring Assessment of peripheral tissues and urine output Titrate in accordance with prescribed blood pressure and other haemodynamic parameters Wean slowly

Nitrates isosorbide dinitrate, nitroglycerine	Vasodilates through relaxation of smooth muscle Dilates venous capacitance predominantly but also arterial vessels Decreases preload and afterload Reduces MVO$_2$ because of peripheral vasodilation Increases heart rate	Following cardiac surgery Used to relieve pain of angina pectoris Hypertension ECG changes due to myocardial ischaemia	Dizziness, headaches Nausea and vomiting Agitation and flushing	Administered orally, transdermal or IV. If IV, should be titrated carefully using an infusion pump Correct hypovolaemic states PVC tubing absorbs a large proportion of NTG
Calcium channel blockers e.g. nifedipine, diltiazem, verapamil, amlodipine	Relaxes vascular smooth muscle reducing peripheral resistance and blood pressure Specific agents have different effects, e.g.: Nifedipine (arterial vasodilator) Diltiazem/verapamil (slows supraventricular patterns)	Useful to reduce blood pressure even where there is evidence of myocardial ischaemia Coronary spasm Slow ventricular response to atrial tachycardias		Some have negative inotropic effect which may be detrimental if cardiac output poor Important to be familiar with effects of specific agent prescribed
ACE inhibitors e.g. enalapril, captopril	Inhibits conversion of angiotensin I into angiotensin II Increases loss of Na and H$_2$O Dilates arterial and venous beds therefore reducing blood pressure Reduces preload and afterload and MVO$_2$	Reduces effect of vasoactive mediators activated by CPB Useful in reducing blood pressure and MVO$_2$ May be given orally or IV Chronic heart failure following myocardial infarction		Observe for hypotension initially Hyponatraemia may be a problem Hyperkalaemia may occur if K-sparing diuretic being taken

Table 6.4 Management of haemodynamic problems

BP	PCWP	CO	SVR	Plan
↓	↓	↓	↓	Volume
N	↑	N	↑	Diuretic or venodilator
↓	↑	↓	↑	Inotrope
↑	↑	↓	↑	Vasodilator
↑↓	↑	↓	↑	Inotrope/vasodilator/IABP
↓	N	N	↓	α agent

BP blood pressure; PCWP pulmonary capillary wedge pressure; CO cardiac output; SVR systemic vascular resistance; IABP intra-aortic balloon pump
↑ = increased; ↓ decreased; N = normal; ↑↓ variable
Source: From Bojar (1999), with permission

Table 6.5 Signs of cardiac tamponade

- Cessation of mediastinal chest drainage
- Low cardiac output
- Hypotension
- Tachycardia
- Raised CVP
- Low urine output
- Narrowing of pulse pressure
- Widening of mediastinum on chest X-ray
- Dysrhythmias
- Decreased voltage on ECG
- Electromechanical dissociation

depolarised with a more positive resting membrane potential. Initially this leads to the cells being more excitable and again may manifest itself as ventricular arrhythmias. However, as the extracellular potassium continues to rise, the cell will not completely repolarise and is therefore unable to depolarise again. The development of these life-threatening arrhythmias is usually preventable through attention to post-operative electrolytes, particularly potassium and the prevention of myocardial ischaemia. Potassium levels should be kept higher than normal in the immediate post-operative period and serum levels of 4.5–5.0 mmol/l are usual. Attention to acid–base imbalance, good oxygenation and measures to balance the myocardial oxygen supply to demand will also reduce the likelihood of these arrhythmias influencing the post-operative course. Once the arrhythmia becomes sustained, urgent treatment is required to terminate it.

Life-threatening arrhythmias in the post-operative period, therefore, may develop for a variety of reasons: drug related, autonomic stimulation, alterations in filling pressures and metabolic or electrolyte imbalance. Poor left ventricular function is a risk factor for sudden death in patients who develop ventricular tachycardia (VT), and regular monitoring and proactive management is therefore even more important in these patients. This usually necessitates closer observation of haemodynamic, respiratory and electrolyte parameters, and will be facilitated by an ICU bed. Fortunately, sustained ventricular tachycardia or ventricular fibrillations, although associated with a poor prognosis, are seen infrequently in the post-operative period (Rho *et al.* 2000).

Atrial arrhythmias may also impact on the post-operative management of the patient following cardiac surgery. Atrial fibrillation (AF) is the most commonly reported, occurring in approximately 30% of patients, with a peak incidence between 2 and 3 days (Kern 1998). It accounts for significant morbidity and prolonged hospital stay while contributing significantly to health cost expenditure. Although a common arrhythmia, and often well tolerated (Riley 2002), for the person following cardiac surgery it may have serious haemodynamic consequences. The loss of atrial contraction may significantly reduce ventricular filling, resulting in reduced cardiac output and blood pressure.

Various causes for AF have been postulated and there is wide agreement that these include:

- Manipulation of the heart tissue
- Cardiopulmonary bypass
- The use of cardioplegic solutions
- Cross-clamping of the aorta
- Hypoxia
- Electrolyte disturbance
- Hypovolaemia
- Sudden increases in left ventricular pressure

It may therefore be assumed that beating heart surgery, avoiding CPB and cardioplegia will result in less AF. Early results have supported this, demonstrating that the incidence of post-operative AF may be as low as 14–21% in patients undergoing off-pump CABG (coronary artery bypass grafting), compared with an estimated 30% in on-pump surgery (Maglish *et al.* 1999; Stamou *et al.* 2000).

Attempts should be made to terminate the arrhythmia if there is evidence of haemodynamic compromise. Cardioversion with drug therapy such as amiodarone is usually attempted and, if unsuccessful, direct current (DC) cardioversion may be used.

If AF persists beyond 48 hours, the risk of thrombotic emboli is increased and anticoagulation (unless contra-indicated) should be commenced. Identifying those at risk of developing AF for prophylactic measures may therefore be successful in reducing the development of this common arrhythmia and the prolonged hospital stay.

The pre-operative use of beta blockers or anti-arrhythmics such as amiodarone may be effective in reducing the post-operative incidence of AF and may help to maintain the ventricular rate, thus reducing the likelihood of a significantly reduced cardiac output (Rho *et al.* 2000). However, even with this prophylaxis, 22% of patients following cardiac surgery may develop AF.

Heart blocks or bundle branch blocks are an unusual complication of the post-operative period, yet when they do occur are frequently associated with myocardial ischaemia. However, during valve surgery, there is an increased risk of a temporary disruption to the atrioventricular (AV) node and Bundle of His due to surgical trauma and oedema. When haemodynamic compromise occurs, or if it is suspected that the heart block will deteriorate, temporary pacing should be considered.

Sinus tachycardia is more likely to be a compensatory mechanism for any low cardiac output, hypovolaemia or be caused by agitation or pain. The first decision in the management of a sinus tachycardia, therefore, is to try to establish and treat the cause.

Bradyarrythmias are more commonly encountered following valve replacement or repair, although with the increased use of beta blockers for the person awaiting revascularisation, they may become more common. The optimal heart rate for ventricular filling is around 100 bpm and therefore bradyarrythmias require urgent treatment. Temporary pacing wires are frequently inserted intraoperatively, when bradyarrythmias are suspected, and these should be used to increase the heart rate. Alternatively, a bradycardia may be treated pharmacologically, for example with intravenous atropine or isoprenaline.

Pacing wires are not routinely inserted, although are more common following valve surgery or when arrhythmias are suspected. When present, the usual practice is for the surgeon to have inserted the pacing wire (either one or two) into the epicardial surface of the right atrium. The end of the wire is then brought out onto the surface of the chest wall. Additional right ventricular wires are sometimes inserted. These wires remain unattached and the ends should be covered with tape and secured to the chest wall. When the patient demonstrates signs and symptoms of haemodynamic compromise caused by a heart block or sinus bradycardia, the end of the wires should be attached to a temporary pacing box.

Epicardial pacing wires are useful in the immediate post-operative period to speed up bradyayrrthmias or to treat symptomatic AV conduction disturbances. However, they will usually become ineffective after about three days. If the arrhythmias persist, a more permanent system should be considered.

Removal of the epicardial pacing wires should be undertaken with care. They are a potential source of infection and should be removed as soon as they are no longer required and certainly before the person leaves the hospital. Using an aseptic technique, the wires should be gently pulled until they slide out. If any resistance is felt, it is wise to cut the wire close to the chest wall and so avoid unnecessary trauma to the heart. When the patient is on anticoagulation, as is common following valve surgery, an International Normalised Ratio (INR) should be checked before the pacing wires are removed. If below 2.5, the pacing wires can be removed. Following the removal of pacing wires the patient should be monitored to eliminate the development of a cardiac tamponade or any arrhythmias. This does not mean that they should remain in a hospital bed, but it is unwise to remove pacing wires on the day of hospital discharge.

Neurological issues

Neurological impairment may occur due to a variety of pre-operative, intraoperative or post-operative factors. These include: atheromatous tissue detaching from the ascending aorta or aortic arch during surgical manipulation; atheromatous debris; micro-bubbles of gas or fat; fibrin–platelet complexes; low perfusion pressures; arrhythmias; and mural wall thrombi. Susceptibility is increased in people with diabetes, carotid artery stenosis, pre-operative heart failure or an enlarged left atrium, and as the trend to operate on the more elderly person increases, the risk of adverse cerebral outcome is likely to increase.

The incidence of post-operative CVA is variable with some studies suggesting it may be as high as 5% in patients undergoing revascularisation, 9% in patients over the age of 75 years and nearly 16% in patients undergoing valvular surgery (Hogue *et al.* 1999). However, the risk of cognitive dysfunction is more common and possibly as high as 80% (Arrowsmith *et al.* 2000). Symptoms include a loss of memory or attention and a decrease in the speed of motor and mental responses. Although these have been frequently described as short term, improving after a few months, more recent work suggests that this cognitive dysfunction may persist (Arrowsmith *et al.* 2000; Newman *et al.* 2001). It is expected that with an increase in beating heart surgery and the avoidance of CPB, a consequent reduction in post-operative neurological dysfunction will be seen (Bhasker Rao *et al.* 1998).

Neurological complications usually become apparent as the patient awakes from the anaesthesia and appears confused, restless or has an apparent neurological deficit. Less commonly, the neurological deficit occurs in the ensuing post-operative period.

Renal dysfunction

The prevalence of renal dysfunction following cardiac surgery may be as high as 35%, although renal failure requiring dialysis is probably much smaller (2–3%) (Morris & St Claire 1999). Many of the factors leading to this serious complication are well known and include low cardiac output, hypovolaemia, CPB and the pre-operative condition of the patient. Hormonal changes associated with major surgery may also adversely affect renal function and include the overexpression of catecholamines, aldosterone, angiotensin and a decrease in nitric oxide secretion (Leme *et al.* 1998). In the period immediately following cardiac surgery, a large diuresis should be expected due to intra-operative haemodilution and this may mask an underlying renal dysfunction.

Close monitoring of urine output alongside maximising cardiac output may either prevent deteriorating renal function or facilitate its early recognition. When suspected, the cardiac output and filling pressures should be maintained and a loop diuretic such as ferosemide administered in the first place. Frequently a low dose of dopamine (1–2.5 mcg/kg/min) is given intravenously. The renal effects of a low-dose of dopamine have received recent interest and the debate continues. Some suggest that the renal effects of dopamine are due to an increase in cardiac output, whereas others suggest that a low dose has a vasodilatory action upon the renal vasculature (Leme *et al.* 1998). Whichever is the true reason, it is clinically apparent that urine output tends to increase following the institution of a dopamine infusion and this remains current practice.

If renal dysfunction appears several days following cardiac surgery, acute tubular necrosis is unlikely and alternative causes such as sepsis or a low cardiac output should be considered.

Gastrointestinal complications

Gastrointestinal (GI) complications, although uncommon, are found in around 0.2% of patients undergoing cardiac surgery. However, they are associated with a high mortality of around 25% (Lazar *et al.* 1995). Several risk factors have been identified and include advancing age, emergency surgery, post-operative inotropic support, poor cardiac function, prolonged CPB or post-operative ischaemia. As the trend towards operating on higher-risk patients continues, GI disturbances are likely to become more common. Predictive modelling to identify those at higher risk of developing such complications may therefore be useful. Acid prophylaxis in the post-operative phase may reduce some risk, while those in higher-risk groups may benefit from gastric pH monitoring. Early oral feeding may also help eliminate some of the problems related to increased gastric acid secretion and so decrease the incidence of post-operative GI complications. Astute assessment skills to recognise those at risk, detect symptoms and initiate early treatment may reduce morbidity, mortality and prolonged hospital stays.

Occasionally a transient ileus develops following prolonged periods of post-operative sedation, analgesia or immobility. Characterised by abdominal bloating, vomiting and absent bowel sounds, a nasogastric tube should be inserted and suction applied. Rarely do these same symptoms relate to abdominal ischaemia which, if present, would be accompanied by extreme abdominal pain.

Although it appears to be well established that poor diabetic control increases the risk of post-operative infections, there has been little clinical research undertaken and little established advice regarding the control of post-operative glucose levels. More recently a study assessing the impact of glucose levels within the first 36 hours following cardiac surgery has demonstrated that when blood glucose levels are higher than 12 mmol/l there is an increase in post-operative complications (Golden *et al.* 1999). As insulin secretion is decreased by CPB while the stress response increases blood glucose levels, it is not unusual to control post-operative blood glucose with intravenous insulin, even in the non-diabetic population.

Vascular complications

Deep vein thrombosis (DVT), the formation of a thrombus in one of the deep veins of the body, more commonly arises in the leg veins, and surgical patients may be at risk for at least six weeks post-operatively (Scurr 1988). Unfortunately for some, the presence of a DVT may lead to pulmonary embolism and death. On the positive side, DVT is frequently preventable through nursing interventions. Using Virchow's triad of predisposing factors, including trauma, blood coagulation and venous stasis, it is apparent that, following cardiac surgery, the patient is at high risk for the development of DVT. The following may all contribute to increased risk:

- Trauma: localised trauma and direct vascular damage caused by vein stripping, intravenous cannulation, intravenous fluid or antibiotic administration

■ Blood coagulation factors: dehydration due to pre-operative nil-by-mouth status, fluid shifts and CPB. Half-heparinisation during off-pump surgery
■ Venous stasis: immobility, low cardiac output, decreased venous return

When present, the signs and symptoms of a DVT include abnormal swelling, warmth, localised pain, pyrexia and colour change of the affected limb but are often difficult to detect when the saphenous vein has been harvested. It is therefore important to identify those at high risk of DVT and use appropriate prophylactic measures. These may include: heparin; pre-operative, intra-operative and post-operative anti-embolism stockings; and physiotherapy with early mobilisation. Only in higher-risk groups should longer-term anticoagulation therapy be considered.

If anti-embolism stockings are to be used they should be carefully fitted with the correct size. For example, where the thigh circumference is greater than 84 cm, below-knee stockings should be used. As compression of the leg arteries may occur it is also necessary to ensure that there is no evidence of peripheral arterial disease (Coppola 1997). If patients are to be discharged home with these stockings then they must be shown how to wear them correctly as inaccurate use has been highlighted as a major area of concern (Peters 1998).

Other vascular complications may occur. Following coronary artery bypass grafting with the saphenous vein, chronic venous insufficiency may result in an increased risk of venous leg ulcers. Although this is a long-term complication of surgery it is worthwhile to suggest the use of venous compression stockings at an early sign of venous ulcer formation or following a cut, bruise or trauma to the leg.

Specific care issues following thoracic surgery

Following thoracic surgery where a thoracotomy has been performed it is usual for the trachea to be extubated as soon as the patient is self-ventilating, arterial blood gases are within normal limits and the level of consciousness is acceptable. A small subgroup of patients may require a period of mechanical ventilation to optimise recovery from what is often an extensive surgical procedure. However, the avoidance of sedatives and mechanical ventilation helps to maintain func-tional residual capacity and minimises the risk of atelectasis. Once transferred to the high-dependency unit (HDU) and haemodynamically stable the patient is nursed sat upright or in a high side lying position. Impaired gas exchange fol-lowing thoracic surgery due to V/Q mismatch can last for as long as 4–6 weeks in some. Table 6.6 outlines some of the complications which may arise following thoracic surgery.

This section initially focuses on pulmonary factors, but additional problems post-thoracotomy may include:

■ Phrenic nerve weakness/paralysis
■ Recurrent laryngeal nerve damage
■ Prolonged air leak which can contribute to surgical emphysema
■ Upper extremity neuromuscular dysfunction due to lateral thoracotomy

Table 6.6 Complications following thoracotomy

Potential problems	Possible changes	Causes	Possible action	Further reading
Hypotension	Fall in BP, tachycardia, JVP ↓ Peripheries cool and pale Diaphoresis Capillary refill >3 s Excessive bleeding via drains (>150 ml/h over 2–3 hours) Possible ↓ haematocrit Possible disorientation Urine output <0.5 ml/kg/h Possible mediastinal shift	Displaced sutures/clips Overt/covert bleeding Haemothorax Dysrhythmias, e.g. atrial Myocardial ischaemia Cardiac failure Bronchopleural fistula Tension pneumothorax Herniation of heart (pericardial approach)	Colloid to maintain CVP within defined parameters Oxygen (FIO_2 0.40) Inotropic agent if necessary Anti-dysrhythmic agents Correct any coagulation problem Tension pneumothorax necessitates chest tube or large-bore needle Re-exploration in theatre to stem any bleeding If broncho-pleural fistula then bronchial closure necessary Correct electrolyte imbalance particularly post-pneumonectomy	Amar 1997 Gothard & Kelleher 1999
Deteriorating pulmonary status/respiratory failure	Tachypnoea/tachycardia Poor chest excursion Vital capacity <15 ml/kg Tidal volume <5 ml/kg Using accessory muscles Falling SpO_2 Diminished breath sounds, wheezes or crackles ↑CO_2 – warm extremities with flapping tremor Restlessness/disorientation Abnormal blood gases	Atelectasis Pneumonia Pneumothorax Broncho-pleural fistula Pulmonary oedema COPD/asthma Acute lung injury (ALI) Acute respiratory distress syndrome (ARDS) Surgical emphysema affecting airway	Reposition to reduce distress (perfusion ↑ through dependent lung – keep any diseased lung uppermost – except pneumonectomy when healthy lung uppermost). Generally, nurse upright/high side lying to increase FRC Check integrity of drainage system Oxygen (FIO_2 0.40), intermittent CPAP, check acid-base status Maintain PaO_2 >8.5 kPa, $PaCO_2$ <6.5 kPa, SpO_2 >92% Deep breathing/expectoration (provide pain relief) Mini-tracheostomy Fluid intake <30 ml/h to avoid over-hydration Bronchodilators/antibiotics Sit out on 1st day and gradually mobilise to avoid complications Mechanical ventilation needed for refractory hypoxaemia	Kilger et al. 1999 Mahamid 2000 Slinger 1995 Orfanos et al. 1999

Pain	Tachycardia, BP↑↓, restless Worsening pulmonary parameters Nausea and vomiting Incisional pain Chest drains Consider non-surgical cause Frozen shoulder on affected side	Continuous analgesic cover, e.g. epidural with bupivacaine and fentanyl. Epidural may result in urinary retention Observe for opiate-induced respiratory depression (early and late) Naloxone should be available to reverse opiate Patient controlled analgesia Regular pain assessment/evaluation Complementary strategies Paravertebral block or patient controlled analgesia	Cheever 1999 Kavangh *et al.* 1994
Infection	Pyrexia >38°C Wound inflammation, pain and discharge Empyema Purulent sputum Inflammation around insertion of vascular lines Exogenous and endogenous factors responsible Poor nutrition, malignancy, elderly, problems with microcirculation etc.	Prophylactic antibiotics given. A cephalosporin is often given peri-operatively plus metronidazole in tracheal resection and oesophagectomy Sputum and wound cultures taken where necessary Appropriate antimicrobial dependent upon sensitivity Address patient local and environmental factors which promote healing	Deschamps *et al.* 1999 Hunt & Williams 1997 Gould 2001 Rai & Dexter 2001

Many patients requiring thoracic surgery have been smokers and inevitably there will be some effect on mucociliary clearance. In addition, fluid restriction and anaesthetic agents can also reduce mucociliary function further. A mini-tracheostomy inserted through the cricothyroid membrane under local anaesthetic may be needed where there is poor expectoration with retained secretions.

Reduced compliance with a restricted pattern of breathing is the norm following thoracic surgery and if resection has been performed then the reduction in lung volume may lead to a fall in effective alveolar ventilation. Ventilatory drive may not be adequate to maintain $PaCO_2$ within normal limits. Hypercapnia may therefore develop post-operatively and confusion, warm extremities, bounding pulse and flapping tremor may all be signs of possible carbon dioxide retention.

Following thoracotomy for resection several predictable changes occur in the intrathoracic cavity where lung tissue has been removed. The remaining healthy lung tissue expands, there is a mediastinal shift towards the operated side and the diaphragm on this side becomes elevated. Following pneumonectomy the space initially fills with blood, fibrin and air, and later with inflammatory exudate. Air absorption from the space is usually complete at six weeks and the space shrinks.

Air leaks post-operatively can be problematical and following resection are usually due to air escaping through small damaged bronchioles and alveoli. Underwater seal drainage is often effective in reducing risk of complications. Air leaks may persist for several days, however, and additional intervention may be required. A major complication following thoracic resection, which is becoming less common, occurs due to the inadequate closure or infection of the bronchial stump. A bronchopleural fistula results and a persistent air leak with cough, haemoptysis and fever. This will necessitate surgical re-exploration and repair.

Hypoxaemia is common following thoracotomy and nursing interventions in the early post-operative phase are aimed at promoting effective pulmonary function and preventing compromise. As soon as the patient is conscious no time is lost in commencing physical therapy with frequent position changes, to aid chest expansion, V/Q relationships and mobilisation of secretions. Following pneumonectomy some surgeons may prefer the patient to be nursed with the operated lung in the dependent position to avoid fluid bathing the bronchial stump with infected secretions and possibly entering the healthy lung.

Haemodynamic status

Hypotension

Hypotension may occur as the patient recovers from the anaesthetic and vaso-dilation occurs with a fall in peripheral resistance. A colloid is usually given and it is usual to give an artificial plasma expander if the haemoglobin is satisfactory, with central venous pressure guiding the volume transfused. Bleeding may be responsible for hypotension and, although this may be overt loss through chest drains, the nurse should be vigilant for signs of covert haemorrhage. Where a drain is not inserted, for example following pneumonectomy, there can be significant blood loss into the chest cavity. Blood loss through drains should be monitored carefully. Loss greater than 2 ml/kg/h over 2–3 hours warrants further investigation including chest radiography, haematocrit and clotting screen. In order to restore blood pressure, vasoactive agents may be needed and the patient's urine output measured hourly. With persistent hypotension a pulmonary flotation catheter may be necessary to assess filling pressures and further surgery may be indicated to stop any bleeding and to evacuate clots.

Cardiac dysrhythmias

Cardiac dysrhythmias are not uncommon following thoracic surgery with 9–33% of patients affected (Amar 1997), and supraventricular arrhythmias, especially atrial fibrillation, are the most common. Many factors are likely to contribute to their development but they occur more frequently in those patients who are older, have a history of cardiovascular disease or following a pneumonectomy or oesophageal surgery. Although atrial tachycardia will respond to resolution of the precipitating factor, other atrial arrhythmias may require pharmacological treatment or cardioversion.

Hydration needs

Following thoracotomy clear fluids are reintroduced several hours following extubation and on the first post-operative day a light diet, if tolerated. The patient's usual oral medication can be recommenced. An intravenous infusion supplies fluid and electrolytes until such time as fluids are taken freely. For the first 48 hours following thoracic surgery care must be taken to ensure that the patient is not fluid overloaded. Altered lung mechanics and the release of inflammatory mediators following resection can result in excessive fluid in the interstitial space because of reduced lymphatic drainage. The risk of this occurring is increased following pneumonectomy and in patients with a history of cardiovascular disease. Because of this, total fluid balance is usually manipulated so that no more than 20 ml/kg of fluid is given during the first 24 hours following surgery.

The patient who has undergone oesophagectomy will probably have thoracotomy and laparotomy incisions. Nutritional difficulties pre-operatively may increase risk for this patient substantially. Because of the anastomosis, care should be exercised when moving to ensure that there is no sudden traction. A nasogastric tube may be inserted following oesophageal surgery and left in position for up to 48 hours. Fluid intake is recommended when bowel movement is confirmed. Confirmation that the oesophagus has healed may be sought by introducing contrast medium and observing for leaks. On no account should the nurse attempt manipulation or reinsertion of the tube following resection as this may cause damage to any anastomoses. Nutritional difficulties may be encountered following oesophageal resections and enteral or parenteral feeding needed. Where diet is poorly tolerated, time should be taken to educate the patient to ensure that dietary habits are adopted which facilitate the passage of food, and follow-up will be necessary to monitor nutritional status.

Thoracic surgery may be needed to treat a variety of disorders although malignancy is probably the most common. However, the patient's diagnosis, specific surgery performed, possible co-morbidity and pre-operative condition will all need to be taken into account to plan and deliver appropriate care in the post-operative period. Following surgery the nurse works closely with the physiotherapist to ensure that pulmonary function is optimised and that return to full mobility achieved without undue delay. With encouragement, the patient is usually able to sit out on the first post-operative day and walk around the bed, with stair climbing often possible on the third or fourth day. Although a persistent air leak may necessitate leaving drains in position longer, early mobility is still important for these patients.

Interventions to optimise pulmonary function following cardiothoracic surgery

A number of measures may be taken to reduce the risk of pulmonary complications in the post-operative period. Ongoing observation of the patient's respiratory rate/depth, chest excursion and distress may alert the nurse to developing problems. An important goal is to increase mobilisation as soon as possible for this will improve circulation, increase lung volumes and prevent complications. Until this is possible, however, there is increased risk, and ongoing pulmonary assessment is crucial. Refer to Fig. 6.2 earlier and note some of the clinical parameters to be monitored. Also note how the initial hypoxaemia can develop into acute ventilatory failure when muscles eventually fatigue.

Pulse oximetry, which measures oxygen saturation, can be a useful tool to monitor trends in pulmonary status. Each molecule of haemoglobin has four binding sites to carry four oxygen molecules. With PaO_2 values within the normal range, saturation should be almost 100%. Because of the shape of the oxyhaemoglobin disassociation curve, even with a PaO_2 of 8 kPa, saturation remains around 90%, but lower than this and saturations drop dramatically, offering no safety margin. Therefore there should be concern when saturations fall below 95% although a lower reading may be acceptable with chronic pulmonary disease. The proportion of haemoglobin combined with O_2 depends on PO_2, irrespective of the amount of haemoglobin present, so while it is useful in detecting hypoxaemia due to poor gaseous exchange it offers little information about oxygen content. So if the haemoglobin were to fall to a low level such as 7 g/dl post-operatively, so long as pulmonary status was satisfactory then saturations would be high – but overall oxygen content low. For example,

$$\text{Content} = \frac{98}{100} \text{ (Sats)} \times (1.39 \times 7) \text{ (plasma } O_2 \text{ omitted)} = 8.3 \text{ ml/dl}$$

Arterial oxygen content should be around 19.5 ml/dl, so in this example the supply side is low and if demand increases (as it does post-operatively) then cellular hypoxia can quickly develop.

Once the patient has been transferred to the ward, with pulse oximetry there should be no need to perform regular arterial blood gas analysis. If there is concern, however, over the patient's deteriorating pulmonary status and saturations are falling, then arterial blood should be drawn to determine acid–base status. A degree of acid–base imbalance is usual following cardiothoracic surgery. Retention of carbon dioxide with an increase in $PaCO_2$ resulting in a respiratory acidosis is often due to hypoventilation where alveolar ventilation is reduced. Following both cardiac and thoracic surgery ventilatory failure may develop in the spontaneously breathing patient due to pain, sedation and/or poor positioning.

The development of acute hypercapnia with respiratory acidosis also results in hypoxaemia which can be life threatening and oxygen therapy is crucial. This is very different from chronic hypercapnia which develops in, for example, neuro-muscular disorders and diseases such as chronic obstructive pulmonary disease. Patients with such chronic ventilatory failure develop long-term compensatory mechanisms including elevated bicarbonate levels. A degree of hypoxaemia is tolerated fairly well in these patients. Respiratory decompensation can occur, however, where there is infection, oversedation or where a high concentration of oxygen is delivered. Management will depend on the cause but the PaO_2 is usually maintained at around 8 kPa while attempts are made to reduce the $PaCO_2$. Patients with chronic hypercapnia may be considered suitable for surgery but there is greater risk of peri-operative complications and mortality. Although mechanical ventilation in chronic ventilatory failure is avoided because of difficulties with weaning, it will become necessary if hypercapnia and acidosis worsen.

When oxygen delivery is impaired with resulting tissue hypoxia, as in low cardiac output states, the accumulation of lactic acid (>2 mmol/l) as a result of anaerobic metabolism results in a metabolic acidosis. Oxygen delivery may be impaired due to a range of factors both pulmonary and circulatory in origin. It is important to remember that following cardiothoracic surgery oxygen demand will be increased because of increased metabolism and excessive protein break-down and the development of a catabolic state will also occur with acidosis (Mitch *et al.* 1994).

If acidosis is not corrected then cardiopulmonary status may be compromised further with decreased cardiac output and arterial blood pressure (Orchard & Kentish 1990), the development of arrhythmias and decreased hepatic and renal blood flow. Acidosis will also increase sympathetic arousal although the effects of catecholamines on the heart and blood vessels will be weakened (Adrogue & Madias 1998), possibly decreasing the effectiveness of some inotropic drugs. Where there is an increase in hydrogen ions, particularly in metabolic acidosis, potassium tends to leave the cells and the resulting hyperkalaemia may have additional adverse effects on the myocardium.

Respiratory alkalosis caused by mild hypocapnia may be permitted following cardiac surgery in the early post-operative period. This mild respiratory alkalosis:

- Decreases respiratory drive
- Allows for the increased carbon dioxide production which will occur during rewarming
- Compensates for possible metabolic acidosis which may have developed because of difficulties with peripheral perfusion

However, more severe respiratory and metabolic alkalosis can have a deleterious effect on cardiopulmonary status.

Oxygen therapy

Supplementary humidified oxygen is usual to correct hypoxaemia for the first 24 hours following extubation in cardiac patients and sometimes for several days following thoracic surgery. A hypermetabolic state post-operatively increases oxygen consumption and delivery must keep up with this increased demand. In cardiac surgery the patient is often cooled, and hypothermia will reduce oxygen requirement initially but, with shivering during the early recovery process, oxygen requirements can increase by up to 300% (Ralley *et al.* 1988).

Oxygen therapy may be delivered through either low (variable performance) or high (fixed performance) flow masks and an FIO_2 of 0.4–0.6 is prescribed. High flow systems provide all the inspired gas (around 40 l/min) and the FIO_2 is not affected by the patient's breathing pattern. These devices result in a high stream of oxygen which entrains room air giving a fixed concentration in the mask reservoir. In the post-operative period a high-flow humidified system is used and there are a number of commercial devices available which, at 10 l/min for example, will provide 40% oxygen. High-flow fixed-performance masks are particularly useful for giving a low accurate FIO_2 in COPD to avoid hypercapnia. In these patients who have a history of type II respiratory failure, initial FIO_2 may be 0.24–0.28 and the aim is to raise the PaO_2 slightly without causing an increase in hydrogen ions (because of hypercapnia). However, in severe hypoxaemia a higher FIO_2 may be prescribed.

A low-flow mask, such as a Hudson mask, does not operate on the same principle and if used with a flow rate of less than 5 l/min can result in significant rebreathing of exhaled air. However, with a flow rate of between 6–10 l/min a concentration of up to 60% can be given. Adding a reservoir bag to the mask can increase this further and the flow rate must be high enough to keep the bag inflated during inspiration. Nasal cannulae are low-flow devices, but in a less acute situation may be a convenient way to administer oxygen which need not be humidified (Table 6.7).

In practice, prescriptions for oxygen are often inappropriate and supervision poor during administration. The doctor should prescribe the oxygen concentration to be given, although in an emergency the nurse must be able to use a system that will effectively reduce hypoxaemia. Oxygen systems should be checked regularly as disconnection can occur. The response to oxygen therapy post-operatively needs to be carefully monitored by oximetry and arterial blood gases. Central cyanosis may be an unreliable sign of tissue hypoxia as it is seen with a reduced haemoglobin concentration of 1.5 g/dl and is often absent in hypoxaemic patients with anaemia (Bateman & Leach 1998). Therapy should be continued until satisfactory saturations are sustained continuously on room air (Gothard & Kelleher 1999).

Cardiothoracic surgery results in a great deal of discomfort, and good pain relief is essential as chest discomfort will result in reduced tidal volumes, hypercapnia and hypoxaemia. If the patient is in pain they may not be able to

Table 6.7 Oxygen administration devices

Fixed performance (High-flow system)	Variable performance (Low-flow system)	Humidified system
Venturi mask	Nasal cannulae	Large-volume nebulisers
2 l/min 24%	1 l/min 24%	5 l/min 28%
4 l/min 28%	2 l/min 28%	8 l/min 35%
8 l/min 35%	3 l/min 32%	10 l/min 40%
15 l/min 60%	4 l/min 36%	
	Hudson mask	
	5–6 l/min 40%	
	6–5 l/min 50%	
	Intersurgical mask	
	2 l/min 28%	
	8 l/min 35%	
	10 l/min 40%	

cooperate with nursing interventions and physiotherapy and there is a danger that secretions will be retained.

Physiotherapy

Although physiotherapy following abdominal and thoracic surgery is beneficial (Fagevik Olsen *et al.* 1997), its efficacy following cardiac surgery is inconclusive. A vital capacity of at least 15 ml/kg is needed to facilitate effective post-operative deep breathing and coughing (Shapiro *et al.* 1991). 'Huff' coughing against an open glottis increases flow rates and may promote more effective clearance of secretions from peripheral airways. However, cough impairment following cardiac surgery need not necessarily result in clinically significant consequences where excessive sputum is not a problem (Stiller *et al.* 1994; Smith & Ellis 2000).

It is the nurse who is present at the bedside all the time and who must remain vigilant in ensuring that chest and limb exercises are performed; her collaboration with the physiotherapist is crucial. A balance needs to be achieved, however, to also ensure that sleep is possible, and coordinating activities of all members of the team to achieve this objective is important and takes persistence and tact.

Breathing exercises are a key component in the post-operative period and deep breathing and expectoration is encouraged. In at-risk cardiac patients, interventions shown to be effective in promoting airway clearance include upright positioning (Dunstan & Riddle 1997), forced expiration technique (Hasani *et al.* 1994) and ambulation (Jenkins *et al.* 1990; Orfanos *et al.* 1999). The active cycle of breathing (Fig. 6.3) is a technique which has been shown to be effective and incorporates breathing control, thoracic expansion and forced expiration techniques (Pryor & Webber 2002). Forced expiratory techniques, however, can sometimes lead to alveolar collapse with worsening hypoxaemia and there must be ongoing evaluation, both during and following treatments. The nurse can

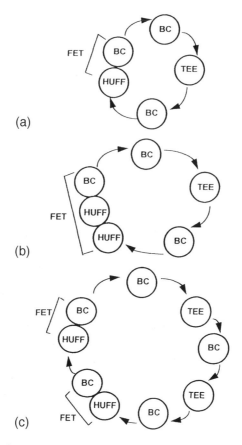

(a)

(b)

(c)

Fig. 6.3 Example of an active cycle of breathing: BC breathing control; TEE thoracic expansion exercise; FET forced expiration technique. Reprinted from Pryor & Prasad (2002), with permission from Elsevier Science.

modify technique to meet the needs of individual patients where, for example, by omitting forced expiration, further pulmonary compromise is avoided.

The use of incentive spirometry following cardiac and thoracic surgery is controversial. It is a technique which encourages voluntary deep breathing by using visual feedback (Wait 1996), yet some studies have shown no difference between incentive spirometry and deep breathing exercises. While there may be some benefit to be gained in high-risk patients this has not been proven in the routine use of incentive spirometry following thoracic procedures (Weiner *et al.* 1997; Gosselink *et al.* 2000). Where there are excessive secretions and wheeze, a bronchodilator such as nebulised salbutamol may be useful.

Patients are often aware of the increased respiratory effort needed during the early post-operative period and may be reluctant to perform physical therapy. Sedation and pain will add to their reluctance. Continuing reassurance and time taken to explain all procedures will encourage, motivate and gain the patient's cooperation.

Additional ventilatory support

Some patients may fail to respond to all attempts to increase pulmonary function and PaO_2 and SaO_2 may continue to fall with the possible development of acute respiratory failure. There are a number of reasons why this may occur, including:

- Worsening atelectasis or lobar collapse
- Nosocomial pneumonia
- Pulmonary oedema (cardiogenic or non-cardiogenic)
- Bronchospasm
- Pre-existing pulmonary disease
- Pneumothorax/haemothorax
- Pulmonary embolism

Hospital-acquired pneumonia is the second most common hospital-acquired infection (George 1996). It is more common in surgical patients than are wound infections (Barie 2000) and the risk for patients following cardiothoracic procedures is particularly high.

Where acute respiratory insufficiency manifests itself, additional respiratory support may be needed. Previously these patients would have been reintubated and positive pressure mechanical ventilation established. There are inherent risks attached to this, however, often resulting in prolonged hospitalisation and increased mortality. The application of non-invasive ventilatory support using a mask or similar device avoids the use of a tracheal tube, laryngeal mask or tracheostomy and is being used increasingly in patients who require ventilation but in whom intubation is not justified.

Continuous positive airway pressure (CPAP)

CPAP is increasingly used in a number of clinical settings to correct hypoxaemia. Positive pressure is applied to the airway via mask, mouthpiece, endotracheal or tracheostomy tube throughout both inspiration and expiration in a spontaneously breathing patient. Flow generators can deliver 50–80 litres of oxygen and air each minute achieving a selected oxygen concentration of between 35% and 90%. More recent non-invasive ventilators may have a CPAP mode, otherwise a high-pressure oxygen supply is needed for the CPAP generator. It is useful post-operatively to improve PaO_2 and saturations by increasing FRC and recruiting previously collapsed alveoli. This latter effect is similar to positive end expiratory pressure (PEEP) used in patients who are mechanically ventilated. In addition, the effects of CPAP in terms of reducing preload and afterload may be beneficial (Mahamid 2000). Not all patients however are able to tolerate CPAP and swallowing of air can lead to gastric distension with vomiting and aspiration. Careful monitoring of patient response is important with checks made on respiratory rate and effort, SpO_2 and haemodynamic parameters. Because the mask needs to fit securely, the condition of the skin should also be checked occasionally. Compared with NIPPV (see below), CPAP in the stable patient does not reduce the work of breathing to the same degree (Elliot *et al.* 1994).

Non-invasive positive-pressure ventilation (NIPPV)

In patients who are hypoxaemic and/or hypercapnic but who are haemo-dynamically stable, alert and cooperative, NIPPV may be appropriate; it comprises the provision of ventilatory support through the upper airway using a mask or similar device. Conventional ventilation utilises a tracheal tube, laryngeal mask or tracheostomy which bypasses the upper airways. Studies which have measured the impact of NIPPV in post-surgical populations are few and samples are often small. Attempts have been made to compare the effects of NIPPV and CPAP in patients with acute cardiogenic pulmonary oedema. In one group (Hoffman & Welte 1999), NIPPV showed an improvement in pulmonary indices with no adverse haemodynamic effects, although in another (Mehta *et al.* 1997), NIPPV was not as effective as CPAP possibly due to increased thoracic pressure, decreased venous return and reduced myocardial perfusion. Caution may need to be exercised where NIPPV is used in patients showing haemodynamic instability.

It is sometimes difficult to wean patients from mechanical ventilation following surgery particularly where there is a history of COPD, and it is here where CPAP and NIPPV may be useful. NIPPV has been successfully used following CABG (Gust *et al.* 1996; Matte *et al.* 2000) and transplantation (Kilger *et al.* 1999). Results have included shorter duration of mechanical ventilation, reduced need for reintubation, reduced nosocomial pneumonia, improved arterial PO_2, and earlier discharge. Even following lung resection, where there is a danger of pleural air leaks due to positive pressure, NIPPV has been shown to improve gaseous exchange without adverse effects (Aguilo *et al.* 1997). In applying NIPPV for acute respiratory failure in the peri-operative setting, careful patient selection and the skill of the team are important if the need for intubation and associated complications are to be avoided (Simonds 2001). The duration of NIPPV varies but treatment is often intermittent allowing treatments to be given and the patient to eat. In the early phases of treatment, however, the patient should be ventilated for as many hours as is clinically indicated and can be tolerated (Kramer *et al.* 1995).

The use of NIPPV is a rapidly developing area reflected in the variety of ventilators available. Both pressure- and volume-cycled models are available and various modes of ventilation possible. Bi-level assisted spontaneous breathing ventilators are often used post-operatively. Inspiratory positive airway pressure (IPAP) facilitates inspiration and a lower expiratory positive airway pressure (EPAP) recruits underventilated lung units. Because of the range of ventilators available, the British Thoracic Society Standards of Care Committee (2002) recommends that one single model of ventilator be used in any one clinical area for ease of training and familiarity of staff with the equipment. Bi-level pressure support ventilators are simpler, cheaper and more flexible than other types available. Once NIPPV has been established, ongoing observation of the patient should include assessment of:

- Chest wall movement
- Coordination of respiratory effort with the ventilator
- Accessory muscle recruitment
- Heart rate

- Respiratory rate
- Patient comfort
- Mental state

Chest drainage

Following cardiothoracic surgical procedures patients will invariably have chest drains inserted. In open heart surgery, drainage and decompression of the mediastinum, pericardium and sometimes pleural cavity (if entered) is required, the primary goals being removal of blood and fluid to prevent cardiac tamponade (short term) or constrictive pericarditis (long term) and prevention of clinically significant pleural effusions (Lancey *et al.* 2001). Suction of around -20 cm is often applied to encourage drainage. Chest tubes or drains are also used after minimally invasive cardiac surgery.

During thoracotomy, as the surgeon enters the thoracic cavity atmospheric air enters the pleural cavity and the chest wall recoils outwards and the lung tissue recoils inwards collapsing. A drainage tube inserted in the pleural cavity facilitates drainage and re-expansion of the lung on the operated side and apical and basal drains are often used. Chest tubes with additional holes allow not only apical removal of air but also basal drainage of fluid. This avoids having to use two separate apical and basal drains.

Chest tubes are usually attached to a sterile underwater seal chamber (2 cm below water level), allowing a one-way valve, so that on expiration fluid and air are removed but on inspiration no air can enter. In pleural chest drainage, this will restore the subatmospheric pressure in the pleural cavity needed for lung expansion. The column of water in the drainage system will 'swing', rising with inspiration as intrathoracic pressure becomes more negative and falling with expiration. This will be reversed if the patient is on a ventilator so that on inspiration with a positive intrathoracic pressure the column will fall and during expiration the column will rise. Continuous suction at around -10 to -20 cmH$_2$O may be applied to facilitate early expansion and reduce bleeding and air leak. Although a one-drainage-bottle system is often used, two bottles allow air to be removed from the apical drain and fluid from the basal drain.

In some patients following thoracic surgery a passive pleural drainage system has been used eliminating the need for connection to wall suction and thus aiding mobility and even discharge home (Johansson *et al.* 1998). Such a system is useful when an air leak persists. A Heimlich valve is a small device allowing air and fluid to be removed on expiration yet the rubber valve prevents air entering the pleural cavity.

Clamping of chest drains should be avoided even during the patient's transfer, as this can be dangerous if an air leak is present. Air will rapidly accumulate in the pleural cavity and result in a tension pneumothorax. Drainage following thoracic surgery results in intermittent bubbling of water in the drainage bottle. Continuous bubbling in a patient self-ventilating denotes an air leak and this is also common following surgery. Checking the system and determining whether any air leak is a new or worsening problem should be initial steps.

Following a pneumonectomy the surgeon may choose not to use chest drainage, and air is aspirated from the pneumonectomy space at the end of surgery. This prevents the mediastinum moving away from the operated side which would otherwise compress the heart and healthy lung, seriously compromising pulmonary and haemodynamic status. If a chest drain is inserted then this should be unclamped for one minute each hour to avoid mediastinal shift; suction should never be applied.

The presence of chest drains adds to the patient's discomfort in the early post-operative period often resulting in severe deep, visceral pain as well as the discomfort caused by the incision. This will further restrict mobility, and efforts must be made to limit the discomfort experienced by the patient. Unfortunately there is a lack of data regarding appropriate interventions in this area. Some studies suggest that even where patient-controlled analgesia is used, patients still experience significant pain (Owen & Gould 1997; Fox *et al*. 1999). Furthermore it appears that pre-operative information regarding chest drainage is lacking and that this may result in reduced effectiveness of analgesic regimens. More intervention studies are needed to determine the most appropriate protocols regarding patient preparation for chest drain and effective use of pain control regimens.

The major focus of research into chest drains has been on suction and the ritual of milking/stripping, although there has been limited research in other areas (Gordon *et al*. 1995). There is scant evidence regarding the benefit of one drainage system over another and practice is based on local policy, often anecdotal and sometimes contradictory.

The drainage system should be secured so that this does not pull and cause discomfort and as much of the system as possible should be visible so that frequent checks can be made without disturbing the patient. Excessive loops in the tubing should be avoided as this will also affect drainage. Tape can be used to secure connections but it would seem sensible to use this in such a way that the join can still be seen. There is no agreement on the type of dressing to use at the insertion site, with many units preferring an occlusive dressing left in place unless soiled. Drainage is recorded regularly and if excessive (>100 ml/h) reported to the medical staff. It is suggested that drainage bottles are changed only when necessary to avoid breaking the circuit and increasing the infection risk. However, as bottles fill with fluid the resistance to drainage increases (Munnell 1997). When a change is necessary, suction should be stopped, the chest drain double-clamped close to the insertion site and the new bottle connected as speedily as possible.

Stripping and milking

Stripping and milking of drainage tubes remains controversial, with one small study (Lim-Levy *et al*. 1986) showing no difference in total drainage and a larger study (Pierce *et al*. 1991) showing significant increase when compared with a control. This technique is not required for apical drains following thoracic surgery which are only removing air. If milking/stripping is required for basal pleural drains, or mediastinal and pericardial drains following cardiac surgery then this should be done gently using only a short section of tube at a time. Stripping the entire length of tube in one manoeuvre can generate pressures of up to

$-400\,cmH_2O$ (Duncan *et al.* 1987). Of the few studies comparing stripping to milking most report no significant difference in outcome (Isaacson *et al.* (1986) *n* = 204; Pierce *et al.* (1991) *n* = 200).

Removal of drains

Drains are removed when drainage is minimal after cardiac surgery or when drainage is minimal (<10-20 ml/h), the lung expanded and any air leak has stopped after thoracic surgery. Before removal the surgeon may request that the tube be clamped for a period to check that lung inflation is complete. Analgesia protocols for drain removal vary widely. In a retrospective audit of chest drain practice in a specialist cardiothoracic centre, 56 different combinations of analgesia were reported by nurses (*n* = 266) and 22 by doctors (*n* = 35), with 10 nurses and 4 doctors giving no analgesia prior to removal (Parkin 2002). Undoubtedly, removal of chest drains is extremely painful and following careful assessment of each individual patient an appropriate analgesic should be administered, although evidence regarding choice is inconclusive.

Removal of a chest drain is usually performed with the patient performing a Valsalva manoeuvre at the end of either inspiration or expiration (Bell *et al.* 2001). The former is often preferred as it is felt that this minimises the risk of air entering the pleura. Close observation of the patient is necessary during and following the procedure as a Valsalva manoeuvre can result in some haemodynamic disturbance. The purse string suture inserted at the time of the drain is secured on its removal and an occlusive dressing usually applied.

Fluid and electrolyte changes following cardiothoracic surgery

In the immediate post-operative period there is often dramatic movement of both fluid and electrolytes across the various fluid compartments particularly following cardiac surgery with cardiopulmonary bypass. Ensuring that fluid and electrolyte balance is maintained will assist in optimising cardiac and pulmonary function. If prescribed fluid replacement is not carefully administered and accurately documented then severe fluid and electrolyte disturbance can occur, with fluid overload and possible oedema (Edwards 2001).

Following cardiac surgery a urinary catheter will be inserted to assist in the monitoring of fluid balance. Hourly urine measurement is important ensuring that all urine is emptied from the drainage tube before each measurement is taken and recorded. Fluid weight gain is to be expected following cardiopulmonary bypass and an osmotic diuresis is usual, although any developing oliguric trend (<0.5 ml/kg/h) should be reported to the medical staff. Not all patients following thoracic surgery will have a urinary catheter. However, if an epidural has been inserted for pain relief then urinary retention may develop, particularly in patients with prostatism, and catheterisation will therefore be needed. Once the epidural has been removed, then so also is the urinary catheter.

Fluid balance in the healthy individual

An understanding of normal fluid balance and the possible changes that can occur as a result of cardiothoracic surgery will assist the nurse in being proactive in both preventing and detecting possible fluid and electrolyte problems post-operatively.

Total body water makes up approximately 60% of body weight in men and 50% on average in women (Fig. 6.4). In a 70kg adult male the total body water is 42 litres and this is distributed as follows:

- Intracellular compartment   28 litres
- Extracellular compartment   14 litres

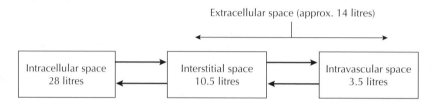

Fig. 6.4   Fluid compartments – total body water approx. 42 litres.

Most of the water, almost two-thirds, is found inside the cells of the body. The above extracellular fluid compartment can be further divided into intravascular (3.5 litres) and interstitial (10.5 litres) compartments (Gabrielli & Layon 1995). The interstitial fluid bathes the cells and any excess fluid is removed by the lymphatic system and returned to the circulation. Body composition changes significantly with advancing age and the percentage of water decreases (Bailes 2000).

The constant movement of fluid across these three compartments enables many different substances to be exchanged between the external environment and the internal milieu ensuring homeostatic balance. Despite huge variations in the extracellular compartment the intracellular compartment is able to remain relatively stable. Starling's forces govern the movement of fluid between the intravascular and interstitial compartments:

- Hydrostatic pressure in the capillaries
- Hydrostatic pressure in the interstitial space
- Oncotic pressure in the capillaries
- Oncotic pressure in the interstitial space

The hydrostatic pressure gradient between the capillaries and the interstitial fluid pushes fluid out of the intravascular space and into the interstitium. Proteins, such as albumin, in the capillary blood plasma and in the interstitium provide an osmotic pressure gradient exerting an osmotic pressure, which is also called oncotic pressure. Lymphatic drainage results in a hydrostatic pressure in the interstitium which prevents excessive accumulation of fluid. In low-albumin situations and increased capillary hydrostatic pressure, fluid can accumulate in the interstitium. This can lead to the development of oedema and increased transcellular water in, for example, the pleural, pericardial and peritoneal cavities.

With outward force from the capillaries usually being slightly greater than the inward force, it is probable that there is a small lymph flow of around 20 ml/h from the pulmonary interstitial space under normal conditions (West 2000). If interstitial fluid volume increases then there is a danger of the alveolar membranes rupturing causing alveolar oedema. One of the most common causes of pulmonary oedema which cardiothoracic nurses encounter is cardiogenic in origin where, due to left ventricular failure there is a rise in left ventricular end diastolic pressure, which is transmitted back to the pulmonary veins (giving an elevated pulmonary capillary wedge pressure, PCWP). This results in an increased capillary hydrostatic pressure with an increase in outward pressure.

Conversely, pulmonary oedema may be non-cardiogenic where the alveolar capillary membrane becomes more permeable, as in acute lung injury because of extracorporeal circulation. Another cause of non-cardiac pulmonary oedema is where there is a decrease in plasma oncotic pressure favouring fluid movement out of the capillaries, as in some renal disorders where there is proteinuria. Figure 6.5 outlines the factors leading to accumulation of fluid in the interstitium resulting in alveolar flooding.

Several abnormal states therefore may promote excessive accumulation of fluid in the pulmonary interstitium.

The exchange of fluid between the intracellular and extracellular compartment is also influenced by the osmolarity, which is the number of dissolved particles per litre of solvent, e.g. water, and is expressed as milliosmoles (mOsm).

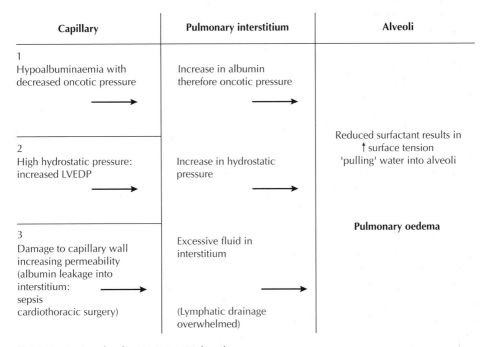

Capillary	Pulmonary interstitium	Alveoli
1 Hypoalbuminaemia with decreased oncotic pressure $\longrightarrow$	Increase in albumin therefore oncotic pressure $\longrightarrow$	
2 High hydrostatic pressure: increased LVEDP $\longrightarrow$	Increase in hydrostatic pressure $\longrightarrow$	Reduced surfactant results in ↑ surface tension 'pulling' water into alveoli
3 Damage to capillary wall increasing permeability (albumin leakage into interstitium: sepsis cardiothoracic surgery) $\longrightarrow$	Excessive fluid in interstitium $\longrightarrow$ (Lymphatic drainage overwhelmed)	**Pulmonary oedema**

Fig. 6.5 Factors leading to interstitial oedema.

Osmolality is the term used when referring to dissolved particles per kilogram of solvent. The value gives an indication of the degree of concentration or dilution of a solvent and, depending on this, water will move across body-fluid compartments by osmosis. In health, the osmolarity of intracellular and extracellular fluid is the same and is around 285 mOsm/l.

The plasma osmolarity is determined by three main solutes – sodium, glucose and urea – but because sodium is the major determinant of plasma osmolarity, doubling the serum sodium value gives a quick approximation. Although water may pass through the semipermeable membranes of the different compartments these solutes usually do not. In a hyper-osmolar state (increased solutes in plasma), water will leave the cells resulting in the cells shrinking; in a hypo-osmolar state the opposite will occur, with water entering the cells (Toto 1998).

The primary electrolytes found in the cell are potassium and phosphate, and in the extracellular compartment sodium and chloride. Although sodium moves between the intravascular and interstitial spaces it does not move quite so freely into the cells. When the serum sodium concentration is low, water moves from the extracellular into the intracellular compartment. Sodium, potassium, glucose and urea are important solutes in plasma which are excreted by the kidneys to maintain acceptable levels across the fluid compartments. In health, the absolute minimum urine output needed to cope with excretion of these solutes is 0.5 ml/kg/h. However, in the critically ill there is often impaired ability of the kidneys to concentrate urine, together with sodium and water retention. Not only is the hourly volume of urine important in assessment, but also the adequacy of urine flow in terms of the amount of solute to be excreted (Gosling 1999). Furthermore, giving too much sodium in replacement fluids post-operatively may result in severe overload.

A number of physiological mechanisms exist to regulate normal electrolyte and fluid balance. The renal system is important in regulating fluid balance and works in concert with the neuroendocrine system to achieve this. If the glomerular filtration pressure in the kidney is low, as in hypotension, then sodium and water reabsorption is increased. The renin–angiotensin–aldosterone mechanism is important in this respect. Both renin and aldosterone are increased following cardiothoracic surgery and these effects can further compromise haemodynamic status.

The antidiuretic hormone (ADH) synthesised in the hypothalamus and stored in the posterior pituitary is released in response to hypovolaemia and increased serum osmolality (e.g. increased sodium). The effect of ADH is to cause water reabsorption, but without sodium and following surgery dilutional hyponatraemia is quite common with low serum osmolality and high urine osmolality.

Post-operative observations

Simple observations such as dry skin and tongue may be indicative of fluid depletion but are quite crude estimates. Diuresis should be observed and this is considered adequate at 0.5 ml/kg/h. Observation of haemodynamic parameters may also alert the team to depletion in intravascular volume, and heart rate, blood pressure, urine output, central venous pressure and pulmonary artery wedge pressure are all useful in monitoring intravascular volume. Generally, a patient with warm skin and good capillary refill has an adequate circulating volume but in some conditions, such as sepsis, blood flow is redistributed to the peripheries at the expense of other vital areas. It is important to remember that inotropic support drugs, by causing vasoconstriction, may suggest haemodynamic stability even though intravascular fluid may be inadequate.

Observing trends in electrolytes is important, as disruption is inevitable due to the effects of surgery. Evaluation of fluid status should be ongoing and involve repeated clinical assessment of sensible and insensible losses (water loss through lung and skin). Insensible loss through the lungs and skin is normally around 600–1200 ml/day but this may be greatly increased because of patient and ambient temperature, humidity, catabolism and high minute volumes. Fluid loss may be underestimated in the high dependency/critical care environment and therefore ongoing observation and recording of losses is crucial.

Post-operatively, patients are in a hypermetabolic, catabolic state and there is often redistribution of fluid and electrolytes from the extravascular space to the 'third space' which includes interstitial, body cavities and intracellular spaces. This is usually increased following cardiac surgery because of an increase in capillary permeability promoting fluid shifts to the third space. Intra-operatively, despite the surgical stress response, blood volume may be maintained by vaso-constriction and neurohormonal factors, but dehydration, hypovolaemia, circu-latory collapse and sepsis can result in huge fluid changes particularly to the interstitial space. In the post-surgical patient, however, any compensatory action to maintain volume may be less effective because renal function is depressed as a result of anaesthetic agents, hypotension and opioids. Spinal and epidural anaesthetics as well as positive-pressure ventilation can all decrease renal blood flow (Gabrielli & Layon 1995).

Interventions to maintain fluid balance post-operatively are therefore aimed at meeting the increased fluid requirements due to fluid movement to the interstitial space.

Fluid replacement

Despite activation of neurohormonal mechanisms following surgery potentially increasing fluid in the interstitium, maintenance of intravascular volume is essential in ensuring adequate preload, left ventricular diastolic volume and therefore optimising stroke volume and renal perfusion. An inadequate intra-vascular volume is associated with hypotension, decreased oxygen delivery to the peripheral tissues and hypoperfusion of essential organs (Kavanagh *et al.* 1995).

The type of fluid selected depends on what needs to be replaced, for example:

■ Red cells to increase oxygen delivery
■ Coagulation factors to reduce risk of bleeding
■ Volume to increase the intravascular space
■ Volume to fill the interstitial space

There is still some controversy remaining regarding the most appropriate fluid to use post-operatively and a recent Cochrane Study (Alderson *et al.* 2003) has compared the effectiveness of colloids and crystalloids in different patient groups.

Crystalloids

Fluids administered usually have the same electrolyte concentration that matches the interstitial fluid (isotonic). Crystalloids are solutions containing electrolytes with a large percentage of water and, because they are isotonic, approximately 75% of the infused volume moves into the extravascular space with half the volume lost within a short time following administration. Crystalloids that contain sodium are the most commonly used replacement fluids to manage post-operative fluid shifts and include normal saline 0.9% which is isotonic and, although containing slightly more sodium than extracellular fluid, does not usually affect tonicity. These fluids rapidly restore the fluid lost from the interstitial space.

Too great a sodium load, however, can increase serum osmolality and through osmosis draw water from the cells, resulting in intracellular dehydration. For this reason, 5% dextrose is often alternated in fluid regimens (Rooney 1995). Many exercise caution when using dextrose solutions in the absence of diseases influencing glucose metabolism, as these preparations do not contain electrolytes and can result in either increased water with dilutional hyponatraemia, or hyperglycaemic hyperosmolarity (Rosenthal 1999). The latter can result in osmotic diuresis and cerebral acidosis. Similarly, hypotonic fluids used to replace the loss of isotonic fluids can quickly result in cerebral oedema and convulsions.

To avoid excessive sodium loads, normal saline is often alternated with a solution such as lactated Ringers or Hartmanns which provide a balanced salt solution. These solutions, however, contain potassium, and careful monitoring of serum potassium is important particularly in patients with renal impairment.

Fluid replacement must be administered cautiously. Following general surgery a maintenance fluid administration of approximately 1–2 ml/kg/h post-operatively meets insensible fluid losses and minimal obligatory urinary losses and it is suggested that it is more detrimental to under- than to over-resuscitate with fluids. However, following thoracic surgery involving resection, it is usual to administer no more than 20–30 ml/kg of fluid in the first 24 hours, and in cardiac surgery 40 ml/kg, with prescribed fluid totals including any losses during the intraoperative period. Following pneumonectomy, pulmonary oedema may develop during the early post-operative period with signs of respiratory distress, and the nurse should be alert to this possibility. Where cardiopulmonary bypass has been used, the peripheral vasodilation that occurs during rewarming may necessitate the administration of additional fluids to maintain an adequate cardiac output.

Colloids

In theory, where there is low intravascular colloid oncotic pressure, the administration of either synthetic agents such as the gelatins, starches and glucose polymers or natural agents such as albumin, plasma protein fraction or fresh frozen plasma can be raised. These agents are given because of their ability to stay in the intravascular compartment for much longer and to facilitate the movement of water back into the intravascular compartment. Colloids, however, do not increase oxygen-carrying capacity nor do they supply clotting factors and because of increased intravascular volume can worsen heart failure. Following surgery, particularly cardiac, endothelial dysfunction due to the systemic inflammatory response may result in increased colloid loss from the vascular compartment. Colloid administration is preferred by some because it is felt that the use of crystalloids would lower the colloid osmotic pressure and increase the risk of pulmonary oedema.

Colloids are more expensive but effective in increasing intravascular volume initially in acute situations:

- Albumin 5% (isotonic) or 20% (hypertonic) – adverse reactions reported
- Gelatins
- Colloid starch suspensions – hetastarch and hexastarch
- Dextrans – large glucose polymers (possible anaphylaxis)

Albumin given to patients who have hypoalbuminaemia has been shown to have a number of adverse effects, including end organ function, coagulation, renal and pulmonary function with increased mortality. For this reason, albumin is not recommended for correcting low serum albumin. In the critically ill where there may be leaky capillary endothelial cells, colloid may leak out of the vascular compartment and lead to the development of oedema and hypotension by accumulating in the interstitial space. The resulting peripheral and pulmonary oedema will increase hypoxaemia and decrease oxygen delivery to the tissues. In some patients the administration of colloids may lead to an allergic reaction.

There is a trend towards using crystalloids for fluid management post-operatively rather than colloids, and while some studies have identified benefits (Velanovich, 1989; Schierhout & Roberts, 1998; Alderson *et al.* 2003) others have not. Although crystalloids reduce oncotic pressure, the reduction in blood viscosity may improve urine output with sodium and potassium excretion and also peripheral flow through the microvasculature, improving tissue perfusion.

The use of colloids in some patients has led to greater improvement in haemodynamic variables compared with the use of crystalloids, with increased cardiac index, colloid osmotic pressure, DO_2 and VO_2 (Hauser *et al.* 1980; Appel & Shoemaker 1981). In some cardiac units the use of colloid for hypovolaemia in the immediate post-operative period may be preferred because of the lower volumes needed and the lower sodium load. Because water and sodium loads increase following surgery owing to neurohormonal compensatory mechanisms, the use of crystalloids is viewed by some as reducing the intravascular oncotic pressure thus further promoting greater fluid shifts to the interstitial space.

Fluid challenge

A fluid challenge involves the administration of small volume (200 ml) of fluid with the aim of restoring circulating volume in hypotensive states while noting carefully the haemodynamic response to each challenge. Ideally the patient's filling pressures and stroke volume are optimised with an improvement in haemodynamic parameters and renal perfusion. Colloids such as the gelatins and starches are occasionally used following cardiothoracic surgery as they have been shown to result in a reliable increase in plasma volume. A fluid challenge may avoid further use of inotropes, the effects of which can be unpredictable because of different α- and β-receptor activity often with tachycardia and increased myocardial oxygen demand.

Electrolytes

A number of changes can take place in the electrolyte balance and this disturbance may seriously compromise the patient, affecting both cardiac and pulmonary function. Fluid replacement therapy should not be considered in isolation from electrolyte balance. Clinical assessment should alert the nurse, often the first to see laboratory data, to the development of electrolyte problems. Results should be carefully evaluated, and possible symptomatic effects noted. Medical staff should then be notified so that appropriate action can be taken to restore equilibrium. Table 6.8 gives examples of electrolytes which can affect cardiac and pulmonary function.

Pain control following cardiothoracic surgery

Nurses have a pivotal role to play in the relief of pain post-operatively and failure to relieve pain increases risk of post-operative complications and further contributes to the surgical stress response. Traditional surgical approaches in cardiothoracic surgery involve posterolateral incisions and sternotomy of the thorax. Most would agree that these are among the most painful surgical interventions (Kavangh *et al.* 1994) particularly thoracic surgical incisions. Severe pain following thoracotomy leads to shallow breathing, impaired ability to cough and changes in respiratory mechanics (Conacher 1990). It results in splinting of the chest during inspiration with diminished tidal volumes, functional residual capacity, possibly leading to atelectasis with profound arterial hypoxaemia (Puntillo & Weiss 1994; Brooks-Brunn 1995).

Prevention of post-operative pulmonary complications is one of the major goals therefore of post-operative analgesia. Post-thoracotomy patients experience a drop in both FVC and FEV_1 to 25% of pre-operative values on the first post-operative day. Overall, reduction in functional residual capacity is the most important mechanical abnormality affecting pulmonary complications (Craig 1981). This leads to atelectasis because the FRC falls below closing volume (the lung volume at which small airways closure occurs), which causes arterial hypoxaemia. Stasis of secretions also occurs which leads to greater potential for pulmonary infections.

Early control of pain can shape its subsequent evolution, and for many patients this can improve clinical outcome following surgery. Decreasing pain results in greater physical mobility, improved pulmonary function, greater patient satisfaction and reduced periods of hospitalisation following surgery (O'Brien 1995). If the nurse is to gain the patient's full cooperation in performing activities to reduce pulmonary complications it is crucial that effective pain control is achieved. Yet poor pain relief remains a problem, with one study ($n = 110$) showing a high incidence of pain following thoracotomy up to 12 months following surgery (Perttunen *et al.* 1999).

Pain is a complex, multi-dimensional phenomenon and it is important to remember that although tissue injury may be a major cause, other factors such as cultural conditioning, expectations, social contingencies, mood state and perceptions of control may also contribute to the experience of pain (Turk & Okifuji 1999). It is a unique experience and differences in individual patients and in the intensity, quality and meaning of pain will result in major differences regarding the manner in which these initial processes unfold.

Physiology of pain

There are three main theories which help to explain the physiology of pain:

- The specificity theory
- The pattern theory
- The gate control theory

The specificity theory supports the transmission of impulses along sensory fibres to a pain centre in the brain earlier thought to be the thalamus. It is now acknowledged that the thalamus simply acts as a sensory relay station and that many different areas of the brain contribute to the total pain experience. The pattern theory supports the generation of pain impulses in a circuital arrangement in the dorsal horn of grey matter at spinal cord level. It is the gate control theory (Melzack & Wall 1965) which has had perhaps the greatest impact on the development of pain relieving strategies in clinical practice. The focus of this theory is on the transmission of pain impulses from peripheral nociceptors through a gating mechanism in the dorsal horn and modulation of this mechanism via descending inhibitory pathways from the brain.

Pain is initiated by the stimulation of peripheral nociceptors which generate pain impulses which are transmitted along sensory nerves to the central nervous system to be processed in the brain. Chemical, physical and thermal energy activates nociceptors generating action potentials along the sensory pathway. Pain impulses are transmitted along small-diameter A-delta fibres (acute pain) which are myelinated and C-fibres (chronic pain) which are non-myelinated. A-delta and C-fibres result in the release of substance P in the dorsal horn and transmission along larger, myelinated A-beta fibres (transmitting touch impulses) closes the gate to further nociceptive signals. Descending inhibitory tracts also stimulate receptor sites in the dorsal horn to release enkephalins. Opioid receptors exist throughout the central nervous system but large numbers are found in the dorsal horn of the spinal cord and the periaqueductal grey area. Natural ligands for opioid receptors in the body include enkephalins, endorphins and dynorphins. The effects of these opioids are antagonised by naloxone.

Table 6.8 Examples of electrolytes monitored in the post-operative period

Electrolyte	Decreased values	Effects	Increased values	Effects	Management
Potassium 3.5–5.5 mmol/l	<3.5 mmol/l <2.5 mmol/l (severe) Stress Hypothermia Reduced intake Diuretic therapy Rapid correction of hyperglycaemia Adrenal hyper-reactivity	Wide PR interval Prominent U wave T waves flat Dysrhythmias Fatigue Muscle weakness (legs)	>5.5 mmol/l Iatrogenic Cardioplegic solutions Acute renal failure Metabolic acidosis Diabetes K^+-sparing drugs	Depressed cardiac membrane potential Peaked T waves Wide PR interval Wide QRS complex Paraesthesia Muscle weakness Muscle cramps Respiratory failure	*Hypokalaemia:* Oral K supplements or IV KCl 20–40 mmol/l of fluid (**no more than 20 mmol/h**). Check local policy regarding peripheral or central vein administration Check phosphate and magnesium levels *Hyperkalaemia:* 10% CaCl IV Glucose/insulin infusion
Sodium 135–145 mmol/l	<135 mmol/l **ECF volume low**, e.g. excessive diuretics, skin/GI loss, glucocorticoid deficiency **ECF volume normal**, e.g. hypokalaemia, drugs, hypothyroidism and hypopituitarism, syndrome of inappropriate ADH secretion (SIADH) **ECF volume high**, e.g. renal failure, nephrotic syndrome, congestive cardiac failure, cirrhosis, psychogenic causes Signs include dizziness, confusion, weakness and haemodynamic problems		>145 mmol/l Increased intake Dehydration from: fever osmotic diuretics diabetes insipidus diabetes mellitus	Thirst Agitation Dry oral mucosa Dry, furred tongue Poor skin turgor	*Hyponatraemia:* 0.9% NaCl and diuretics for any overload *Hypernatraemia:* Dextrose 5% IV

Magnesium 1.4–2.2 mmol/l	<1.4 mmol/l Inadequate intake Diuretic therapy post-operatively	Atrial and ventricular dysrhythmias Wide QRS complex Peaked T wave ST depression Coronary spasm Delirium/convulsions Muscle weakness	>2.4 mmol/l Excessive administration Renal failure	CNS depression with altered mental state Cardiac toxicity Prolonged PR interval Nausea and diarrhoea Appetite loss Muscle weakness	*Hypomagnesaemia:* Magnesium sulphate 2 g in 100 ml
Phosphorus 0.84–1.45 mmol/l	<0.84 mmol/l Poor dietary intake Post-operative stress Catecholamine induced Increased renal loss in COPD when theophyllines prescribed	Lethargy Muscle weakness/ tremor Cardiac dysrhythmias Decreased diaphragm contraction	>1.45 mmol/l		*Hypophosphataemia:* Intravenous replacement with either sodium or potassium

ECF extracellular fluid

Transmission of pain impulses through the dorsal horn can be inhibited therefore by closing the gate, as in:

- Stimulation of the large-diameter A-beta fibres
- Stimulation of opioid receptors
- Stimulation of descending inhibitory impulses (also stimulating opioid receptors)

There is increasing evidence supporting a 'wind-up' process which occurs following initial nociceptive activity and this intense central nociceptive activity can result in electrophysiological and morphological changes in the dorsal horn (Wall & Woolf 1986) resulting in remodelling (plasticity) within the spinal cord and precipitating long-term chronic pain syndromes. Such pain offers no biological advantage and causes a great deal of suffering and distress. This maladaptive pain resulting from damage to the sensory nerve pathway of the nervous system is known as neuropathic pain and may last longer than six months (Merskey & Bogduk 1994). Even brief intervals of acute pain can induce this long-term neuronal remodelling (Carr & Goudas 1999) and the biological and psychological foundation for long-term persistent pain is in place within hours of injury (Niv & Devor 1998).

Pain as a stressor

Surgical pain is a major stressor and will evoke not only local but general responses also. A hypermetabolic state is initiated and there is an increase in substrate mobilisation and in the rate of biochemical reactions. This is referred to as the stress response, and while adaptive it can also impair recovery through activation of the endocrine, immune and inflammatory pathways.

Pain following surgery can result in adverse physiological responses including the microcirculation which can further compromise oxygen delivery during the post-operative period. The limbic system, as a result of anxiety and fear, communicates with the hypothalamus, driving the classic pituitary–adrenal and sympathomedullary stress responses with increased levels of cortisol and catecholamines resulting in a hypermetabolic state. This response will (Kehlet 1989):

- Increase serum fibrinogen therefore viscosity
- Increase blood glucose and fatty acids
- Increase ADH
- Impair the immune response and wound healing

As well as the above global stress response, massive tissue injury inflicted during surgery also generates high circulating concentrations of cytokines (interleukins, interferon and TNF) released by phagocytic cells and cells of the immune system which also have an important role in the inflammatory process. Interleukins such as IL-1 and IL-6 bypass the brain and act directly on the pituitary to stimulate corticotrophin and vasopressin secretion. This response can profoundly affect the cardiovascular system, with increases in catecholamines and vasopressin causing increased peripheral vascular resistance and blood pressure with increased afterload, stroke volume and cardiac output (Bernauer & Yeager 1993). The resting increased myocardial oxygen demand may further compromise the cardiac patient and additional effects of the stress response may include impaired wound healing, deep vein thrombosis, pulmonary embolism and sepsis.

Pain assessment

An important component of any pain relief strategy is the explanation given to the patient and this should commence before surgery. Patients are concerned, if not fearful, about the pain they will experience. Time must be taken to explore these fears and to reassure the patient that although they will feel discomfort there is much that can be done to relieve their pain. As early as 1964, Egbert and colleagues demonstrated that pre-operative discussion with patients about the surgical procedures and associated discomfort halved the requirement for post-operative analgesia and reduced time to discharge. Nursing studies further endorse that information giving before surgery contributes to better pain relief and results in fewer complications (Hayward 1975; Boore 1978). Indeed, a number of studies have now been carried out which identify the benefits of cognitive and behavioural interventions pre-operatively, including decreased anxiety before and after surgery, reduced post-operative pain intensity and intake of analgesic drugs, improved treatment compliance, cardiovascular and respiratory indices, and accelerated recovery (Kiecolt-Glaser *et al.* 1998).

A number of pain assessment tools are available and whenever possible these should be introduced before surgery. Pain control involves far more than the administration of analgesics and previous experiences of pain and successful personal coping strategies should be documented.

Visual scales can help patients to communicate their pain level and are particularly useful during the acute phase when they are unable to speak. These involve descriptive scales ranging from no pain to worst possible pain, numerical scales from 0 to 10, and a 10 cm visual analogue scale ranging from no pain to worst possible pain. Scales are available for patients with language difficulties (Whaley & Wong, 1989). These scales only measure the sensory component although pain also has affective and cognitive aspects. For useful information on other nursing-related pain issues in cardiothoracic settings, see Hiscock (1998).

As pain transmission involves transduction, transmission, modulation and perception, any pain control strategy should involve recognition of these resulting in 'balanced analgesia' (Boysen & Blau 1995). This is useful when considering pain relief (Fig. 6.6).

With regard to surgical pain, transduction is the process whereby physical and chemical energy generates electrical action potentials at the site of peripheral nociceptors. Multiple interacting mediators and receptors allow for sensory integration and modulation of nociceptive input in the periphery (Carlton & Coggleshall 1998). These chemical mediators, e.g. prostaglandins, bradykinin, substance P – many from inflammatory cells, are capable of stimulating nociceptors. Many mediators that operate at the peripheral site are also operational at

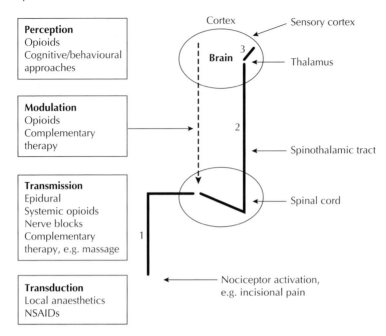

Fig. 6.6   Sites to consider when relieving pain following surgery.

the spinal cord level. Transduction can be targeted, therefore, by an agent that prevents the synthesis of inflammatory mediators at this site and non-steroidal anti-inflammatory drugs (NSAIDs) are often prescribed. Pre-emptive analgesia has been used in an attempt to reduce 'wind-up' and excessive nociceptive activity before pain is experienced and, although benefit has been shown, this is not consistent in all studies. Inhibiting transmission of electrical pain impulses along the sensory pathways is usually achieved by intravenous opioids, nurse-controlled opioid infusions and in thoracic surgery epidural analgesia also. Cryoanalgesia is used infrequently although paravertebral blockade is preferred by some thoracic surgeons.

Pharmacological agents

An important component of any pain control strategy in the peri-operative period is the use of pharmacological agents – non-opioid and/or opioid analgesics. Non-opioids, used for post-operative pain which is mild to moderate include NSAIDs such as diclofenac, keptoprofen, naproxen and ibuprofen. Paracetamol may also be effective for some patients. Intravenous infusion or rectal administration of diclofenac is also sometimes used to prevent the occurrence of post-operative pain.

Opioid analgesics

There are weak and strong opioids and their use in pain control following cardiothoracic surgical procedures is commonplace. A powerful systemic opioid is usually given short term with the patient progressing onto oral medication thereafter. Although the post-operative course for most patients is fairly predictable, and indeed protocol driven, assessment by the nurse should identify those patients who require systemic opioids a little longer. Pain management cannot be considered individualised when all patients have their systemic opioids discontinued routinely after 48 hours.

The effect of any opioid will depend on the morphine receptor site targeted in the central nervous system, e.g. mu-1 receptors (analgesia) and mu-2 receptors (hypoventilation, bradycardia, physical dependency and euphoria). Opioids are preferred in the management of post-operative pain because of several effects, including:

- Modulation of pain at the spinal cord level in the dorsal horn
- Activation of descending inhibitory pathways from the brain
- Mood-elevating effects
- Anxiety reduction

Weak opioid analgesics include codeine phosphate, co-dydramol, co-proxamol and co-codamol and are classified as narcotic agonists. Their analgesic site of action is at the endogenous opiate receptor binding sites. Codeine phosphate is often used in combination with non-narcotic analgesics such as paracetamol for symptomatic treatment of mild to moderate pain. Some of the administered codeine is converted in the liver to morphine, accounting for its mild analgesic properties.

Systemic opioids

Systemic opioids are commonly used following cardiac and thoracic surgery and include agents such as morphine, diamorphine and fentanyl. Fentanyl is a popular opioid because it has weak local anaesthetic properties and enhances the peripheral nerve block analgesic action of local anaesthetics when administered into the epidural space.

Patient-controlled analgesia (PCA)

Intra-operative general anaesthesia and 'as needed' approaches to post-operative pain evoke higher concentrations of stress hormones, more intense pain, more substantial catabolism and greater immune impairment than regional local anaesthetic blockade (Kehlet 1989). Opiates need to be administered in such a way that steady therapeutic levels are maintained. Bolus 'as needed' opioids can result in supra-therapeutic levels with respiratory depression, orthostasis or ileus, and sub-therapeutic levels (Kaier 1992) with increased pain and stress. Patients who cannot use a PCA pump should receive an opioid around the clock by continuous IV infusion with additional bolus analgesic agents before painful procedures (Cheever 1999).

PCA is often used in patients following cardiothoracic surgery and is a technique that allows the patient to self-administer a small intravenous bolus of an analgesic, usually highly potent opioids, at frequent intervals using a special PC pump (Azad 2001). If the patient is able to cope with this method then excellent pain relief can be achieved. Delay is eliminated by the use of a fixed prescription delivered by a microprocessor-controlled pump. Although affording the patient more control, nurses should be alert for signs of opioid-related side-effects such as respiratory depression particularly if a background infusion is used (Ashburn *et al.* 1994). It has been shown, however, that there is no benefit gained from continuous basal drug infusion during PCA.

Not all studies have demonstrated superior analgesia with PCA (Murphy *et al.* 1994; Myles *et al.* 1994). In one study, PCA was compared with nurse-controlled analgesia (*n* = 66) and whereas PCA did not provide superior pain relief compared with nurse-controlled infusion analgesia, patients experienced significantly less nausea (O'Halloran & Brown 1997).

Epidural analgesia

Epidural analgesia following thoracotomy has been shown to provide very efficient pain relief (Azad *et al.* 2000). An opiate administered via a thoracic epidural cannula following cardiac surgery has also shown similar benefits in terms of reduced hormonal stress response and improved pulmonary function (El-Baz & Goldin 1987). Simultaneous administration of opioids and local anaesthetics can moderate the pain response and possibly enhance mediator release blockade. This is particularly true with continuous infusion and works in most patients (Fischer *et al.* 1988), although it is suggested that any benefit from the addition of bupivacaine to fentanyl in thoracic epidural analgesia is confined to the early postoperative period (Mahon *et al.* 1999). There seems to be fewer side-effects with this technique compared with the use of either local anaesthetics alone (hypotension) or opioid alone (pruritus, nausea, potential respiratory depression).

Lipid-soluble opioids such as fentanyl and sufentanil are removed from the cerebrospinal fluid more quickly than morphine, reducing the risk of delayed respiratory depression which can occur with morphine (De Leon-Casasola & Lema 1996). A continuous infusion occasionally causes hypotension, probably due to interference of the cardiac sympathetic supply, although some have shown an overall reduction in post-operative complications with epidural infusions of local anaesthetic agents (Yeager *et al.* 1987). A comparison of PCA with an epidural of fentanyl and local anaesthetic has shown superior pain relief in the epidural group but no difference with regard to pulmonary complications and duration of hospital stay (Azad *et al.* 2000).

Side-effects occasionally seen with epidurals include respiratory depression, oversedation, hypotension, pruritus and urinary retention. Respiratory depression with opioids can occur occasionally, and although this is usually in the first few hours, it can occur much later. The fear of respiratory depression can be exaggerated and this should not result in the withholding of opioids as the incidence of respiratory depression in patients receiving epidural opioids is less than 1% (McCaughey & Graham 1982). Ongoing observation by the nurse is crucial and naloxone should always be at hand for immediate administration should the effects of morphine need to be reversed.

Although the use of epidurals following thoracotomy is a specialised procedure it is integral to acute pain management and, with an appropriate education programme, nurses can provide skilled care in this area (Richardson 2001).

In some patients following thoracotomy the use of extrapleural analgesia may be employed. This involves placing an indwelling catheter in the extrapleural space at the end of surgery. Extrapleural analgesia has been found to give good pain control and preservation of pulmonary function (Richardson *et al.* 1999a). In one study, paravertebral bupivacaine was superior to epidural bupivacaine in terms of pain relief, pulmonary function and side-effects (Richardson *et al.* 1999b). Although some surgeons prefer paravertebral blocks, until this particular method has been evaluated further, epidurals following thoracotomy are likely to be the preferred option.

Following cardiac surgery, epidural anesthesia may be problematical, with an increased risk of spinal haematoma formation (Turfrey *et al.* 1997). With the increase in beating heart surgery and the consequent reduction in the use of heparin, epidural anaesthesia may be used.

Sedation

Pain may not be the major concern of the patient and a great deal of anxiety may be generated by a host of factors in the post-operative period: immobilisation, chest drains and oxygen therapy, for example. Opioids offer some sedation, but because these effects are secondary many believe that sedation should be considered as a separate therapeutic goal (Boysen & Blau 1995), so that in addition to pain assessment, anxiety assessment should also be considered using a visual analogue scale. Although some degree of sedation is usual in the critical care environment, this may still be required for some patients when transferred to the ward. For critically ill patients, benzodiazapines are often used to achieve sedation and anxiolysis, and diazepam, lorazepam and midazolam have been all used with varying degrees of success.

During the course of the patient's post-operative care there may be occasions when additional pain relief is required. For example, removal of chest drains and other invasive devices can be excruciatingly painful for some patients. Nitrous oxide and oxygen (Entonox™) has been used with success for some painful procedures. However, the practice of pain relief at such times varies widely between units, with no pain relief given at all in some cases. Vasovagal episodes have been observed during short painful procedures and further research is needed in order to develop appropriate protocols. Individual patient assessment is important and effective pain relief should remain an important goal.

Non-pharmacological interventions in pain relief

Pharmacological agents feature greatly in cardiothoracic pain relief protocols but there are other non-pharmacological interventions which may also be useful and have the potential to further modulate nociceptor activity, particularly in the dorsal horn. For example, more than 200 studies demonstrate that pre-emptive cognitive and behavioural interventions can decrease anxiety before and after surgery and accelerate recovery (Kiecolt-Glaser *et al.* 1998). Together with more traditional orthodox approaches, non-pharmacological interventions may increase further the effectiveness of pain relief protocols. Work in this area is still in its infancy, but as complementary approaches are becoming more mainstream and as studies are demonstrating their worth, nurses are in an ideal position to develop appropriate interventions for patients following surgery. The effectiveness of specific interventions is likely to be influenced by a host of factors and it is worth remembering that although one particular intervention may not benefit the patient, another may.

Table 6.9 outlines some of the complementary approaches which have been used in cardiothoracic surgery although most studies have involved patients following cardiac surgery. However, some studies have shown positive results in patients following general surgery so some benefit is likely. Once again, more research is needed here.

The mind–body dualism which has dominated orthodox medicine and health care is no longer tenable, and integrated medicine which combines complementary and traditional treatment approaches is the future of health care (Shirreffs 1996). Although there are many studies which claim benefits in different patient groups, the methodology is often lacking. Nevertheless, there have been several systematic reviews carried out investigating the evidence regarding claims made, and indeed benefits have been found. More research is needed involving larger numbers, and funding needs to be made available for this. With increasing evidence and growing public interest, nurses need to be proactive in this area, gaining the appropriate information and skills grounded in scientific inquiry.

Post-operative infection

Infection post-operatively is costly, delays discharge and is responsible for a great deal of distress to patients and their families. The hospital inpatient infection rate is approximately 9%, with surgical wound infections responsible for 10.7% of these (Emmerson 1996). Costs to the country account for approximately £1 billion each year (Plowman 1999). In addition to large surgical wounds, a number of invasive lines will be used either to monitor the patient's progress or to administer various pharmacological agents. *Staphylococcus aureus*, part of the normal flora in the nose, throat, axillae, toe webs and perineum of 30–40% of healthy people in the general population (Gould & Brooker 2000), is the most common cause of pyogenic infection, responsible for about 33% of all hospital-acquired infections (Gould 2001).

The patient undergoing cardiothoracic surgery will be at risk of developing an infection post-operatively because of a number of different factors. The nurse should be knowledgeable regarding these factors so that the local and general environment can be manipulated and all measures taken to minimise the risk. In addition, an awareness of factors promoting health and wound healing will enable the nurse to plan effective care for the patient following surgery.

Before any discussion regarding the risk of infection, a preliminary outline of the principles of wound healing is given.

Table 6.9 Examples of complementary approaches in pain relief

Intervention	Rationale and effect	Patient groups/studies	Additional issues
Transcutaneous electrical nerve stimulations (TENS)	Use of skin electrodes to deliver low-voltage stimulus *Benefits:* Thought to increase endorphins and inhibit transmissions along pain fibres	Thoracotomy (Benedetti *et al.* 1997)	Not for patients with pacemakers/cardiac arrhythmias Only useful for mild to moderate pain post-thoracotomy
Music therapy	Music delivered by headphones Anxiolytic effects well documented *Benefits:* May increase mood and patient tolerance	Used in many settings including: MI (White 1999) CABG (Blankfield *et al.* 1995) chest tube removal (Broscious 1999) during bronchoscopy (Colt *et al.* 1999) (Evans 2002, systematic review)	Inexpensive with few side-effects Little expertise needed Should be used pre/post-operatively Useful in cardiac patients and many other groups
Massage, e.g. feet, back, neck, shoulders Often combined with aromatherapy	Systematic manipulation of soft tissue. *Benefits:* Distraction; improved circulation; reduced anxiety and pain; enhanced immune response; decreased stress hormones; improved sleep	CABG (Stevenson 1994) (Richards *et al.* 2000, systematic review)	Assessment important Recognise cultural and personal feelings Not appropriate for first 48 hours following surgery Individual assessment and evaluation important
Relaxation and guided imagery	Diverting the patient's thoughts to achieve a calm, silent still mind *Benefits:* Reduced stress hormones, physiological arousal, anxiety; earlier discharge following CABG; improved sleep	CABG (Miller & Perry 1990; Halpin *et al.* 2002) (Seers & Carroll 1998, systematic review) (Johnstone & Vogele 1993, meta-analysis)	Audiotapes can be used with pre-recorded narrated stories No evidence that relaxation harmful. Only weak evidence to support effectiveness in acute pain. More research needed

Principles of wound healing

Wound healing is divided into three main phases, inflammation, proliferation and maturation (Cox 1993). Inflammation, the body's non-specific immune response, is initiated at the time of surgery where the surgeon's incision injures the local tissue environment and microcirculation. Many different inflammatory cells, including leucocytes, release cytokines, many of these having both growth-promoting and chemotactic properties. Neutrophil influx is particularly marked in the early inflammatory response, with macrophage and lymphocyte activity occurring a little later (Moore 1999). Platelets are particularly crucial in this respect, releasing platelet-derived growth factor (PDGF).

The proliferative phase initially involves the growth of endothelial cells stimulated by PDGFs and fibroblast growth factor. This angiogenesis is important in the migration of capillary endothelial cells into the wound to establish a source of blood flow to the tissues. Fibroblasts migrate in response to both growth factors and chemo-attractants and have a key role in collagen synthesis. Repair and remodelling of tissue includes the movement and replication of epithelial cells, also under the influence of growth factors. This epithelialisation begins within 24 hours and in a clean surgical wound is generally complete by the third post-operative day (Gould 2001). Finally it is the maturation phase where remodelling continues, governed by fibroblasts and proteases achieving a balance between deposition and degradation (Kingsley 2002). During this phase the wound also shrinks and shortens as collagen fibres are pulled together.

Dressings

There is a huge variety of commercially prepared dressings available to promote healing of surgical wounds and most surgical units have devised local protocols to guide practitioners. Although an absorbent dressing will have been applied in the operating theatre this can usually be removed when bleeding has stopped and the wound is often left open. If a wound dressing is used then this should (Whitby 1995):

- Permit gaseous exchange to maintain PO_2 and pH at appropriate levels
- Maintain high humidity in the area to promote epithelialisation
- Maintain wound temperature close to body core temperature to facilitate mitosis and phagocytosis
- Aid removal of dead tissue and bacterial, chemical and physical contaminants thus preventing bacterial infection and limiting the inflammatory phase
- Be impermeable to bacteria
- Protect healing tissue from disruption by physical forces; be non-adherent, non-allergenic and free from contaminants

Conditions to promote healing

Ideally, wounds following surgery heal by first intention where the above inflammatory response and subsequent phases are effective. For this to occur, however, a number of conditions must be met. Healing and resistance to infection become better as local perfusion and oxygenation improve, so wound care demands attention to local blood supply, respiratory variables and cardiac output, with hypoxia impairing immunity and repair (Hunt & Williams 1997). Any pre-existing condition where the circulation is impaired, e.g. diabetes, may contribute to wound problems. Local tissue oxygen tension and perfusion in the first 48 hours after surgery is related to collagen accumulation several days later, and where there is adequate oxygenation and perfusion more collagen accumulates than in tissues that are poorly perfused (Jonsson *et al.* 1991).

Failure to meet hydration needs will also affect perfusion, and by infusing relatively small volumes the subcutaneous tissue oxygen tensions can be increased. Ensuring adequate infusion of either colloid or crystalloid fluid, therefore, will promote wound healing by increasing peripheral blood flow and oxygen delivery (Hartmann *et al.* 1992). It therefore follows that giving supplementary oxygen in the first 48 hours following cardiothoracic surgery will also influence subcutaneous oxygen tensions, and despite the many variables involved in oxygen delivery it is suggested that arterial saturation levels should remain 94% or more (Whitney & Heitkemper 1999).

Prolonged hypothermia following cardiac surgery may impair healing because of the local vasoconstriction which occurs, and effective rewarming to re-establish a core temperature of at least 36°C will improve local perfusion and healing.

Factors which may affect the microcirculation and therefore oxygen supply to wounds include:

- Hypothermia
- Sympathetic arousal resulting in peripheral vasoconstriction (stress/low volume etc.)
- Administration of sympathomimetic agents
- Smoking history
- Diabetes mellitus

Because of the factors listed, the risk of wound complications is high following cardiac surgery because of the effects on the microcirculation. The next section outlines specific wound problems in cardiac and thoracic surgical patients.

Sternal wounds

The rate of sternal wound infection is between 1.5% and 7.2% and the infection is a major cause of morbidity and increased health costs in adults (Loop *et al.* 1990; Zacharias & Habib 1996). Infection of sternal wounds can be either superficial or deep and result in sepsis and death. In one centre, possible contributing factors were categorised into pre-operative, intra-operative and post-operative (Hussey *et al.* 1998), and this provides a useful guide (see Table 6.10).

People with diabetes have a 2–5 times greater risk of sternal wound infection

Table 6.10 Factors contributing to sternal wound infection/dehiscence

Pre-operative factors	Intra-operative factors	Post-operative factors
Diabetes mellitus	Use of bilateral and single	Hypotension/hypoperfusion
Chronic obstructive	internal mammary artery	Sympathomimetic agents, e.g.
pulmonary disease (COPD)	(IMA)	dopamine/dobutamine
Pre-operative intensive care	Long operative time	Ventilatory support >48 hours
stay	(>4 hours)	Post-operative CPR
Obesity	Long cardiopulmonary time	Reopening of chest
Advanced age (>70 years)	(>2 hours)	Banked blood transfusions
Sex (male)		Hypoxaemia
Cigarette smoking		
Impaired immune response		

than the non-diabetic population (Furnary *et al.* 1999). The degree of risk for sternal wound infection in men and women is not clear. Whereas males are accorded greater risk in some studies (Hussey *et al.* 1998), in others, females have been shown to have increased risk (Stahle *et al.* 1997; Sofer *et al.* 1999). Although many of the factors identified are not amenable to intervention, a knowledge of risk factors for each patient will assist in identifying those most vulnerable. This may then contribute towards early detection and prompt treatment.

The routine use of the internal mammary artery in coronary artery bypass grafting (CABG) may have led to improved patency rates and survival (see Chapter 5), yet also results in damage to the sternal blood supply. This may impede sternal healing and lead to early dehiscence and infection. The risk is greater where both internal mammary arteries are used and still further in the elderly and patients with diabetes (Grossi *et al.* 1991; He *et al.* 1994), although there is a suggestion that any increase in sternal wound breakdown is minimal (Taggart 2002). Damage to the blood supply is caused by cauterisation, and alternative techniques, which involve careful dissection of the internal mammary artery without cauterisation, have reduced the risk slightly (Sofer *et al.* 1999).

Sternal dehiscence, where there is separation of the sutured sternum, can occur with or without infection. Sternal dehiscence without infection usually occurs quite early in the post-operative course, whereas infection occurs later. Infection of the sternal wound may result because of infection elsewhere in the body or because of contamination from some external source.

Superficial sternal infection may simply be associated with local erythema and discharge and respond to appropriate wound care and antimicrobial therapy. Deeper infection should be suspected in the presence of unexplained low-grade fever, leucocytosis, sternal wound tenderness/instability with cellulitis, purulent wound drainage, chest or neck discomfort and malaise, and can appear 2–3 weeks following surgery. With deeper sternal wounds, complications are more common and morbidity and mortality increase as a result. Mediastinitis, for example, arises when there is suppuration of the anterior mediastinal space, and this a serious complication of cardiac surgery, possibly arising in 1–3% of patients (Vaska 1993). It requires early diagnosis and treatment as infection may extend retrosternally to the heart, coronary artery grafts, prosthetic valves and intracardiac sutures with an associated mortality rate of 24–40% (Rosenbaum *et al.* 1990). Involvement of the chest wall can also lead to long-term complications of osteomyelitis and costo-chondritis, with even greater mortality.

Sternal wounds should be inspected daily for signs of redness or drainage and the patient should be advised to do the same once discharged home. Patients should also be advised to seek medical help if they experience persistent pain over the sternal wound site even if apparently healed. Although the pain may occur because of the sternal wiring, it may be a sign of mediastinitis. Stability of the sternum can be assessed through asking the patient to cough while holding a hand firmly over the sternum. Any rocking or clicking may indicate sternal instability and that the sternal bone has not healed. Often this just requires resuturing, although sternal instability may indicate underlying infection.

With deep sternal infection the infective organism should be identified as soon as possible. If there is no wound drainage, then aspiration of the infection should be undertaken. Antimicrobial therapy with an anti-staphylococcal and gram-negative agent is important and is usually prescribed for several weeks. A number of interventions may be necessary to treat a deep infection, including exploration and drainage. A second mediastinotomy is necessary to debride any necrotic or infected tissue and to drain purulent material. The surgeon may request that the wound be left open to facilitate drainage. A catheter may be positioned in the mediastinum to facilitate irrigation (e.g. antibiotic solutions/saline) of the infected cavity over the course of several days. For a number of years iodine was used as a broad spectrum antiseptic but lost favour mainly because of reported patient sensitivity. However, it is suggested that iodine may be suitable for clinically infected chronic wounds and acute management of the surgically drained abscess (Gilchrist 1997). Where sternal debridement, rewiring, closed drainage and irrigation fail or where there is severe infection with involvement of other structures then major debridement and reconstructive surgery may be necessary (Jones *et al.* 1997). In order to encourage wound closure, omentum or muscle flap transposition (using pectoralis major or rectus abdominus) is occasionally performed, and while for many surgeons this is a last resort, it is suggested that reconstructive surgery should be a first-line therapy for deep sternal infection (Brandt & Alvarez 2002).

Infection of the leg wound occasionally occurs owing to problems with the microcirculation as outlined earlier and this is more common in the overweight, diabetic or those with peripheral vascular disease (Utley *et al.* 1989). Inflammation may be due to both infective and non-infective causes. When due to infection then cellulitis with wound breakdown and purulent drainage are usually evident. The wound infection may respond to antibiotics, debridement and meticulous wound care.

Thoracotomy wounds

The vascular problems inherent with cardiac surgical wounds are not usually present with wounds following thoracic surgery. Generally, wounds can be left exposed after 24–48 hours with wound sutures removed after 7–10 days and drain sutures 2–5 days following removal. One of the most common reasons for performing thoracic surgery is malignancy, and these patients are at an increased risk of infection. Although some patients may present with neutropaenia, so long as the leucocyte count is greater than $500/mm^3$ there is usually no problem with wound healing (Schaffer & Barbul 1996). Diabetes, long term steroid therapy, immunocompromise due to any cause and obesity are all important factors.

Empyema

Infection of the pleural space can develop for a number of reasons. Following thoracic surgery it usually occurs after pneumonectomy and partial lung resections and is a serious complication. Cough, purulent sputum, anorexia, weight loss and fever with night sweats are common features. When empyema occurs after pneumonectomy it is often associated with a bronchopleural fistula (BPF) and mortality is significant. Following a lung resection it occurs in 2–16% of patients (Deschamps *et al.* 1999), but as it may occur many years following surgery, the incidence is probably underestimated. Multiple peri-operative factors, both local and systemic, are associated (Deschamps *et al.* 2001) and causative pathogens are usually *Pseudomonas aeruginosa* and *Staphylococcus aureus*. Features indicative of BPF include persistent air leak and in the absence of chest drainage, expectoration of serosanguinous fluid from the post-pneumonectomy space, with possible contamination of the healthy lung and aspiration pneumonitis.

Empyemas may be treated by the insertion of an intercostal drain. However with chronic empyemas this is more difficult. The location of the empyema is identified on a CT (computerised tomography) scan and bronchoscopy is often carried out to exclude a BPF. Treatment of a chronic empyema may necessitate leaving the chest tube in and converting the closed drainage system to an open system. The chest tube is usually cut so that 2–3 cm is left exposed and a safety pin employed to prevent retraction into the cavity. A suture ensures that the tube is anchored and does not fall out. A dressing is applied or an 'ostomy' device used to collect the drainage (Finkelmeier 2000). The tube may remain in position for several weeks, while it is gradually shortened and eventually removed once a sinogram has checked the remaining cavity. Delayed healing with empyema can cause considerable distress for the patient and, as with all chronically infected wounds, can have a devastating effect on body image and self-esteem. Wounds that become chronically infected cause profound disappointment, and any resulting depression can impair further the healing process.

Intravascular catheters

Intravascular catheters are necessary during and following cardiothoracic surgery to monitor physiological parameters and to administer drugs. Infection of these accounts for around one-quarter of nosocomial infections (Rai & Dexter 2001) and can lead to catheter-related bloodstream infection (CRBI). Responsible organisms include *S. epidermidis*, *Staphylococcus aureus* and candida groups, and central venous catheters are particularly susceptible. Staff should remain vigilant for any

signs of local infection – redness, swelling, soreness and discharge. Local protocols should be followed for obtaining cultures for withdrawn catheters and performing diagnostic tests with the catheter still in position.

A number of precautions may avoid the development of intravascular catheter
sepsis and include:

- Maximal aseptic technique for insertion
- Use of gauze rather than transparent dressing (Mermel 2000)
- Avoidance of ointments at insertion site (Mermel 2000)
- Disinfection of hubs and ports (e.g. chlorhexidine) before accessing
- Adequate specialist nurse/patient ratios (Soifer *et al.* 1998)
- Minimal manipulation of catheters (Soifer *et al.* 1998)
- Anticoagulant prophylaxis (Randolph *et al.* 1998)

Localised infection with organisms other than pseudomonas may be treated
with antibiotics without removal of the catheter (Rai & Dexter 2001), but for
systemic infection the catheter should be withdrawn and appropriate antibiotic
treatment started.

Modern health care, although responsible for tremendous improvements in
health, unfortunately is also responsible for the unabating difficulties experienced
with antibiotic resistance. This is a problem facing both hospital and community,
with pathogens developing where conventional antibiotics are ineffective, e.g.
methicillin-resistant *Staphylococcus aureus* (MRSA) and vancomycin-resistant
enterococci (VRE). Prescribing habits involving antibiotics, patterns of health care,
and lack of effective infection control policies and procedures have led to
increased prevalence over the years.

Until the development of new agents to deal with these organisms, prevention
is the major weapon for containing the spread of infection, with hand-washing
perhaps the most effective measure that health professionals can take. Pathogens
commonly causing infections are *Staphylococcus aureus* and *S. epidermidis*. Transient bacteria from the hand may be easily transmitted from practitioner to patient
and this indeed is considered to be the main cause of bacterial spread in health
care settings (Gould 1991).

Decubitus ulcers

The same factors which increase risk for surgical wound infection following
surgery can also contribute to the development of pressure sores. Laying or sitting
for long periods during the early post-operative period for patients who have
been chronically ill and are hypoxaemic and possibly receiving inotropic support
post-operatively, can quickly lead to trauma and devitalisation of tissues.
Ongoing observation and inspection of pressure areas, correct manual handling
procedures and use of pressure-relieving devices will all contribute to reducing
risk.

Despite all preventive methods, some patients will have surgical wounds which
are difficult to heal. Control of odour, exudates and pain is important. Wounds
may need debridement as debris may act as a focus of infection. Materials that

adhere to the wound, such as gauze, are not recommended for routine use. A huge variety of products is now available which promote autolytic wound debridement, including hydrocolloids, hydrogels, polysaccharide beads/paste, foam dressings and alginate dressings as well as bio-surgical techniques (sterile maggots). The choice of dressing for any wound should be considered only after careful assessment. It is not possible to explore this in any great detail here, but Fig. 6.7 offers an example of an algorithm which can be used to aid selection of the most appropriate wound dressing.

Promoting healing

Identifying factors contributing to the healing process and the restoration and promotion of health in the post-operative period should be thought of in both local and global terms. The nurse is in a key position to ensure that the continuity of care is such that conditions are met which optimise this healing process.

Rest and sleep

When we are sleeping there will be approximately 4 to 6 complete sleep cycles. Each cycle consists of four stages beginning with stage 1, which is non-rapid eye movement (NREM) sleep, progressing through stages 2 to 4 and followed by a short period of rapid eye movement (REM). The REM period following the first cycle is quite short, but subsequent periods are more prolonged until eventually stages 3 and 4 (slow wave) of NREM sleep disappear and the REM sleep lasts around 30 minutes. It is during REM or 'dream' sleep that emotional healing, brain restoration and growth occurs, with NREM important for promoting physical healing and growth (Evans & French 1995). Because stages 3 and 4 of NREM sleep occur only during the first two cycles and it is during this stage that cell repair takes place, disturbed sleep can result in impaired healing because of a reduction in growth hormone. Each time the patient is disturbed they must return to stage 1 of the initial sleep cycle.

The healing properties of rest and sleep have been recognised for some time and it is during this restorative process that protein synthesis and cell division occur (Horne 1998). Psychoneuroimmunology has established a link between psychological factors, the immune response and healing (Kiecolt-Glaser *et al.* 1995). Sleep difficulties in patients cared for in acute care settings remain a real problem and can be attributed to environmental noise, pain, discomfort, and not least the constant stream of health care workers around the bedside. The clustering of nursing activities is crucial in order to avoid constant interruption. Following cardiac surgery researchers have demonstrated ($n = 97$) the interaction between noise-induced stress and other stress in predicting poorer patient sleep (Topf & Thompson 2001). Poor sleep and sleep deprivation can also increase anxiety and stress and interfere with the immune system, disrupting the crucial role of macrophages and lymphocytes (Irwin *et al.* 1994). Everything possible must be done, therefore, to provide adequate rest, and it is important that at least 90 minutes of continuous sleep is allowed to ensure one full sleep cycle, the minimum required for healing.

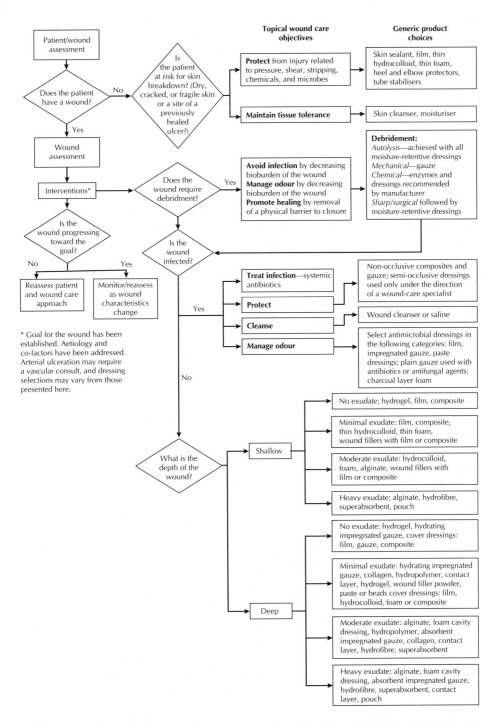

Fig. 6.7 Local wound management interventions algorithm. From Rolstad *et al.* (2000), with permission.

Benefits of a holistic approach

Ideally, surgical wounds should heal by first intention and the skilled nurse will adopt a holistic approach in carrying out a risk assessment and in ensuring that patient, local and environmental factors are addressed to promote wound healing and prevent infection. Once there is an established focus of infection, as well as patient distress, delayed discharge and increased financial cost, the patient is at high risk of developing septicaemia and septic shock, which can result in multi-system failure and death. The nurse is the only health professional to be with the patient throughout a 24-hour period and can do much to influence the post-operative course when the patient is most vulnerable. With forethought and meticulous attention to detail in preventing cross-infection, additional distress, at a time which is already stressful for the patient, can be avoided.

For most patients the post-operative course is relatively uneventful and early discharge possible. Despite the major trauma involved for the patient undergoing cardiac and thoracic surgery, the body has an amazing capacity to deal with this and maintain equilibrium. Skilled, ongoing assessment by the cardiothoracic nurse ensures not only that each patient has the physical, psychological, emotional and social resources to cope but also that appropriate measures are taken when recovery is compromised.

References

Adrogue, H.J. & Madias, N.E. (1998) Medical progress: management of life threatening acid–base disorders – first of two parts. *New England Journal of Medicine* **338**(1): 26–34.

Aguilo, R., Togores, B., Pons, S., Rubi, M., Barbe, F. & Agusti, A. (1997) Non-invasive ventilatory support after lung resectional surgery. *Chest* **112**(1): 117–21.

Alderson, P., Schierhout, G., Roberts, I. & Bunn, F. (2003) Colloids versus crystalloids for fluid resuscitation in the critically ill. *Cochrane Review*. In: The Cochrane Library, Issue 2. Oxford: update software.

Amar, D. (1997) Prevention and management of dysrhythmias following thoracic surgery. *Chest Surgery Clinics of North America* **7**: 818.

Appel, P.L. & Shoemaker, W.C. (1981) Evaluation of fluid therapy in adult respiratory failure. *Critical Care Medicine* **9**: 862–9.

Arrowsmith, J., Grocott, H., Reves, J. & Newman, M. (2000) Central nervous system complications of cardiac surgery. *British Journal of Anaesthesia* **84**(3): 304–7.

Ashburn, M.A., Love, G. & Pace, N.L. (1994) Respiratory related critical events with intravenous patient controlled analgesia. *Clinical Journal of Pain* **10**: 52–6.

Azad, S.C. (2001) Perioperative pain management in patients undergoing thoracic surgery. *Current Opinion in Anaesthesiology* **1491**: 87–91.

Azad, S.C., Groh, J., Beyer, A. *et al.* (2000) Continuous epidural analgesia vs patient controlled intravenous analgesia for postthoracotomy pain. *Acute Pain* **3**: 84–93.

Bailes, B.K. (2000) Perioperative care of the elderly patient. *Association of Perioperative Registered Nurses Journal* **72**(2): 185–207.

Bare El, Y., Ross, A., Kalawi, A. & Egeburg, S. (2001) Potentially dangerous negative intra-pleural pressures generated by ordinary pleural drainage systems. *Chest* **119**(2): 511–14.

Barie, P.S. (2000) Importance, morbidity and mortality of pneumonia in the surgical intensive care unit. *American Journal of Surgery* **179**(Suppl. 2A): 2S–7S.

Bateman, N.T. & Leach, R.M. (1998) ABC of oxygen. Acute oxygen therapy. *British Medical Journal* **317**: 798–801.

Bell, R.L., Ovadia, P., Abdullah, F., Spector, S. & Rabinovici, R. (2001) Chest tube removal: end-inspiration or end-expiration? *Journal of Trauma* **50**: 674–7.

Benedetti, F, Amanzio, M., Cavallo, A. *et al.* (1997) Control of postoperative pain by transcutaneous electrical nerve stimulation after thoracic operations. *Annals of Thoracic Surgery* **63**(3): 608–10.

Bernauer, E.A. & Yeager, M.P. (1993) Optimal pain control in the intensive care unit. *International Anaesthesiology Clinics* **31**: 201–21.

Bhasker Rao, B., VanHimbergen, D., Edmonds, H. *et al.* (1998) Evidence for improved cerebral function after minimally invasive bypass surgery. *Journal of Cardiac Surgery* **13**(1): 27–31.

Blankfield, R.P., Zyzanski, S.J., Flocke, S.A., Alemagno, S. & Scheurman, K. (1995) Taped therapeutic suggestions and taped music as adjuncts in the care of coronary artery bypass patients. *American Journal of Clinical Hypnosis* **37**: 32–42.

Bojar, M. (1999) *Manual of Perioperative Care in Cardiac Surgery*, 3rd edn. Blackwell Science, Oxford.

Boore, J. (1978) *Information: A Prescription for Recovery*. Royal College of Nursing, London.

Boysen, P.G. & Blau, W.S. (1995) Pain management and sedation in the intensive care unit. In: Gallagher, T.J. (ed.) *Postoperative Care of the Critically Ill Patient*. Williams & Wilkins, London.

Brandt, C. & Alvarez, J. (2002) First line treatment of deep sternal infection by a plastic surgical approach: Superior results compared with conventional cardiac surgical orthodoxy. *Plastic and Reconstructive Surgery* **109**(7): 2231–7.

British Thoracic Society Standards of Care Committee (2002) Non-invasive ventilation in acute respiratory failure (BTS Guideline). *Thorax* **57**(3): 192–211.

Brooks-Brunn, J. (1995) Postoperative atelectasis and pneumonia. *Heart & Lung* **24**: 94–115.

Broscious, S.K. (1999) Music: an intervention for pain during chest tube removal after open heart surgery. *American Journal of Critical Care* **8**: 410–15.

Carlton, S.M. & Coggleshall, R.E. (1998) Nociceptive integration: does it have a peripheral component? *Pain Forum* **7**: 71–8.

Carr, D.B. & Goudas, L.C. (1999) Acute pain. *The Lancet* **353**(9169): 2051–8.

Cheever, K.H. (1999) Reducing the effects of acute pain in critically ill patients. *Dimensions of Critical Care Nursing* **18**(3): 14–23.

Colt, H.G., Powers, A. & Shanks, T.G. (1999) Effect of music on state anxiety scores in patients undergoing fibreoptic bronchoscopy. *Chest* **116**: 819–24.

Conacher, I.D. (1990) Pain relief after thoracotomy. *British Journal of Anaesthesia* **65**: 806–12.

Coppola, R. (1997) Chronic venous insufficiency and leg ulceration. *Physician Assistant* **21**(3): 30–36.

Cox, D. (1993) Growth factors in wound healing. *Journal of Wound Care* **2**(6): 339–42.

Craig, D.B. (1981) Postoperative recovery of pulmonary function. *Anaesthesia and Analgesia* **60**: 46.

De Leon-Casasola, O.A. & Lema, M.J. (1996) Postoperative epidural opioid analgesia: what are the choices? *Anaesthesia and Analgesia* **83**: 867–75.

Deschamps, C., Pairolero, P.C., Allen, M.S. *et al.* (1999) Early complications: bronchopleural fistula and empyema. *Chest Surgery Clinics of North America* **9**: 587.

Deschamps, C., Bernard, A., Nichols, F.C. *et al.* (2001) Empyema and bronchopleural fistula after pneumonectomy: factors affecting incidence. *Annals of Thoracic Surgery* **72**: 243–7.

Des Jardins, T., Burton, G.G. & Tietsort, J. (1997) *Respiratory Care Case Studies: The Therapist Driven Protocol Approach*. Mosby, London.

Doering, L. (1997) Relationship of age, sex and procedure type to extubation outcome after heart surgery. *Heart and Lung* **26**(6): 439–47.

Duncan, C.R., Erickson, R.S. & Weigel, R.M. (1987) Effects of chest tube management on drainage after cardiac surgery. *Heart and Lung* **16**: 1–9.

Dunstan, J. & Riddle, M. (1997) Rapid recovery management: the effects on the patient who has undergone heart surgery. *Heart and Lung* **26**(4): 289–98.

Edwards, S. (2001) Regulation of water, sodium and potassium: implications for practice. *Nursing Standard* **15**(22): 36–45.

Elasser, A., Schlepper, M., Klovekorn, W. *et al.* (1997) Hibernating myocardium: an incomplete adaptation to ischaemia. *Circulation* **96**(9): 2920–31.

El-Baz, N. & Goldin, M. (1987) Continuous epidural infusion of morphine for pain relief after cardiac operations. *Journal of Thoracic and Cardiovascular Surgery* **93**: 878–83.

Elliot, M.W., Aquilina, R., Green, M., Moxham, J. & Simonds, A.K. (1994) A comparison of different modes of non-invasive ventilatory support: effects on ventilation and inspiratory muscle effort. *Anaesthesia* **49**: 279–83.

Emmerson, A. (1996) The second national prevalence survey of infection in hospitals: overview of results. *Journal of Hospital Infection* **32**: 175–90.

Evans, D. (2002) The effectiveness of music as an intervention for hospital patients: a systematic review. *Journal of Advanced Nursing* **37**(1): 8–18.

Evans, J.C. & French, D.G. (1995) Sleep and healing in intensive care settings. *Dimensions of Critical Care Nursing* **14**(4): 189–99.

Fagevik Olsen, M., Hahn, I., Nordgren, S. *et al.* (1997) Randomised controlled trial of prophylactic chest physiotherapy in major abdominal surgery. *British Journal of Surgery* **84**: 1535–8.

Finkelmeier, B.A. (2000) *Cardiothoracic Surgical Nursing.* Lippincott, New York.

Fischer, R.L., Lubenow, T.R., Liceaga, A. *et al.* (1988) Comparison of continuous epidural infusion of fentanyl-bupivacaine and morphine-bupivacaine in management of postoperative pain. *Anaesthesia and Analgesia* **67**: 559–63.

Fox, V., Gould, D., Davies, N. & Owen, S. (1999) Patients' experiences of having an underwater seal chest drain: a replication study. *Journal of Clinical Nursing* **8**(6): 684–92.

Furnary, A.P., Zerr, K.J., Grunkemeier, G.L. & Starr, A. (1999) Continuous intravenous insulin infusion reduces the incidence of deep sternal wound infection in diabetic patients after cardiac surgical procedures. *Annals of Thoracic Surgery* **67**: 352.

Gabrielli, A. & Layon, A.J. (1995) Acute electrolyte imbalances in the critically ill postoperative patient. In: Gallagher, J.T. (ed.) *Postoperative Care of the Critically Ill Patient.* Williams & Wilkins, London.

George, D.L.(1996) Nosocomial pneumonia. In: Mayhall, C.G. (ed.) *Hospital Epidemiology and Infection Control.* Williams & Wilkins, Baltimore.

Gilbert, T.B., Barnas, G.M. & Sequeira, A.J. (1996) Impact of pleurotomy, continuous positive airway pressure and fluid balance during cardiopulmonary bypass on lung mechanics and oxygenation. *Journal of Cardiothoracic and Vascular Anesthesia* **10**: 844–9.

Gilchrist, B. (1997) Should iodine be reconsidered in wound management? *Journal of Wound Care* **6**(3): 148–50.

Golden, S., Peart-Vigilance, C., Kao, L. & Brancati, F. (1999) Perioperative glycemic control and the risk of infectious complications in a cohort of adults with diabetes. *Diabetes Care* **22**(9): 1408–14.

Gordon, P.A., Norton, J.M. & Merrell, R. (1995) Refining chest tube management: analysis of the state of practice. *Dimensions of Critical Care Nursing* **14**(1): 6–12.

Gosling, P. (1999) Fluid balance in the critically ill: the sodium and water audit. *Care of the Critically Ill* **15**(1): 11–16.

Gosselink, R., Schrever, K., Cops, P. *et al.* (2000) Incentive spirometry does not enhance recovery after thoracic surgery. *Critical Care Medicine* **28**(3): 679–83.

Gothard, J. & Kelleher, A. (1999*) Essentials of Cardiac and Thoracic Anaesthesia.* Butterworth-Heinemann, Oxford.

Gould, D. (1991) Nurses' hands as vectors of hospital acquired infection: a review. *Journal of Advanced Nursing* **16**: 1216–25.

Gould, D. (2001) Clean surgical wounds: prevention of infection. *Nursing Standard* **15**(49): 45–56.

Gould, D. & Brooker, C. (2000) *Applied Microbiology for Nurses.* Macmillan, London.

Grossi, E.A., Esposito, R., Harris, L.J. *et al.* (1991) Sternal wound infections and use of internal mammary artery grafts. *Journal of Thoracic and Cardiovascular Surgery* **102**: 342–6.

Gust, R., Gottschalk, A., Schmidt, H., Bottiger, B.W. & Bohrer, M.E. (1996) Effects of continuous (CPAP) and bi-level positive airway pressure (BiPAP) on extravascular lung water after extubation of the trachea in patients following coronary artery bypass grafting. *Intensive Care Medicine* **22**: 1345–50.

Hall, R., MacLaren, C., Smith, M. *et al.* (1997) Light versus heavy sedation after cardiac surgery: myocardial ischaemia and the stress response. *Anaesthesia and Analgesia* **85**(5): 971–8.

Halpin, L., Speir, A., CapoBianco, P. & Barnett. S. (2002) Guided imagery in cardiac surgery. *Outcomes Management* **6**(3): 132–7.

Hartmann, M., Jonsson, K. & Zederfeldt, B. (1992) Effects of dextran and crystalloids on subcutaneous oxygen tension and collagen accumulation. *European Surgical Research* **25**: 270–77.

Hasani, A., Pavia, D., Agnew, J.E. & Carke, S.W. (1994) Regional lung clearance during cough and forced expiration technique (FET): effects of flow and viscoelasticity. *Thorax* **49**: 557–61.

Haslam, P.L., Baker, C.S., Hughes, D.A. *et al.* (1997) Pulmonary surfactant composition early in development of acute injury after cardiopulmonary bypass: prophylactic use of surfactant therapy. *International Journal of Experimental Pathology* **78**: 277–89.

Hauser, C.J., Shoemaker, W.C., Turpin, I. & Goldberg, S.J. (1980) Oxygen transport responses to colloid and crystalloids in critically ill surgical patients. *Surgery* **150**: 811–16.

Hayward, J. (1975) *Information: A Prescription Against Pain.* Royal College of Nursing, London.

He, G.W., Acuff, T.E., Ryan, W.H. & Mack, M.J. (1994) Risk factors for operative mortality in elderly patients undergoing internal mammary artery grafting. *Annals of Thoracic Surgery* **57**: 1453–60.

Hebert, P.C., Wells, G., Blajchman, M.A. *et al.* (1999) A multicentre, randomised, controlled clinical trial of transfusion requirements in critical care. *New England Journal of Medicine* **340**: 409–17.

Hiscock, M. (1998) Pain. In: Shuldham, C. (ed.) *Cardiorespiratory Nursing.* Stanley Thornes, Cheltenham.

Hoffman, B. & Welte, T. (1999) The use of non-invasive pressure support ventilation for severe respiratory insufficiency due to pulmonary oedema. *Intensive Care Medicine* **25**: 15–20.

Hogue, C., Murphey, S., Schechtman, K. & Davila-Roman, V. (1999) Risk factors for early or delayed stroke after cardiac surgery. *Circulation* **100**(6): 642–7.

Horne, J. (1998) *Why We Sleep.* Oxford University Press, New York.

Hunt, T.K. & Williams, H. (1997) Wound healing and wound infection. *Surgical Clinics of North America* **77**(3): 587–606.

Hussey, L.C., Leeper, B. & Hynan, L. (1998) Development of the sternal wound infection prediction scale. *Heart and Lung* **27**(5): 326–36.

Irwin, M., Mascovich, A., Gillin, J.C., Willoughby, R., Pike, J. & Smith, T.L. (1994) Partial sleep deprivation reduces natural killer cell activity in humans. *Psychosomatic Medicine* **56**: 493–8.

Isaacson, J.J., George, L.T. & Brewer, M.J. (1986) The effects of chest tube manipulation on mediastinal drainage. *Heart and Lung* **15**: 601–5.

Jenkins, S.C., Souta, S.A., Loukota, J.M., Johnson, L.C. & Moxham, J. (1990) A comparison of breathing exercises, incentive spirometry and mobilisation after coronary artery surgery. *Physiotherapy Theory and Practice* **6**: 117–26.

Johansson, J., Lindberg, C.G., Johnsson, F., von Holstein, C.S., Zilling, T. & Walther, B. (1998) Active or passive chest drainage after oesophagectomy in 101 patients: a prospective randomised study. *British Journal of Surgery* **85**(8): 1143–6.

Johnstone, L. & McKinley, D. (2000) Cardiac tamponade after removal of atrial intracardiac monitoring catheters in a paediatric patient: case report. *Heart and Lung* **29**(4): 256–61.

Johnston, M. & Vogele, C. (1993) Benefits of psychological preparation for surgery: a meta-analysis. *Annals of Behavioural Medicine* **15**: 245–56.

Jones, G., Jurkiewicz, J.J., Bostwick, J., Wood, R., Bried, J.T. & Culbertson, J. (1997) Management of the infected median sternotomy wound with muscle flaps: the Emory 20-year experience. *Annals of Surgery* **225**: 766.

Jonsson, K.J., Jensen, J.A., Goodson, W.H. *et al.* (1991) Tissue oxygenation, anaemia and perfusion in relation to wound healing in surgical patients. *Annals of Surgery* **214**: 605–13.

Kaier, K.S. (1992) Assessment and management of pain in the critically ill trauma patient. *Critical Care Nursing Quarterly* **15**: 14–34.

Kavangh, B.P., Katz, J. & Sandler, A.N. (1994) Pain control after thoracic surgery. *Anesthesiology* **81**: 737–59.

Kavanagh, R.J., Radhakrishnan, D. & Park, G.R. (1995) Crystalloids and colloids in the critically ill patient. *Care of the Critically Ill* **11**(3): 114–19.

Kehlet, H. (1989) Surgical stress: the role of pain and analgesia. *British Journal of Anaesthesia* **63**: 189–95.

Kern, L. (1998) Management of postoperative atrial fibrillation. *Journal of Cardiovascular Nursing* **12**(3): 57–77.

Kheradmand, F., Wiener-Kronish, J.P. & Corry, D.B. (1997) Assessment of operative risk for patients with advanced lung disease. *Clinics in Chest Medicine* **18**: 483–94.

Kiecolt-Glaser, J.K., Marucha, P.T., Malarkey, W.B. & Glaser, R. (1995) Slowing of wound healing by psychological stress. *Lancet* **346**: 1194–6.

Kiecolt-Glaser, J.K., Page, G.G., Marucha, P.T., MacCallum, R.C. & Glaser, R. (1998) Psychological influences on surgical recovery: perspectives from psychoneuro-immunology. *American Psychologist* **53**: 1209–18.

Kilger, E., Briegel, J., Haller, M. *et al.* (1999) Effects of non-invasive positive pressure ventilatory support in non-COPD patients with acute respiratory insufficiency after early extubation. *Intensive Care Medicine* **25**: 1374–9.

Kingsley, A. (2002) Wound healing and potential therapeutic options. *Professional Nurse* **17**(9): 539–44.

Kloner, R., Arimie, R., Kay, G. *et al.* (2001). Evidence for stunned myocardium in humans: a 2001 update. *Coronary Artery Disease* **12**(5): 349–56.

Kochamba, G.S., Yun, K., L, Pfeffer, T.A. *et al.* (2000) Pulmonary abnormalities after coronary arterial bypass grafting operation: cardiopulmonary bypass versus mechanical stabilisation. *Annals of Thoracic Surgery* **69**: 1466–70.

Kramer, N., Meyer, T.J., Meharg, J. *et al.* (1995) Randomised prospective trial of non-invasive positive pressure ventilation in acute respiratory failure. *American Journal of Respiratory Critical Care Medicine* **151**: 1799–806.

Lancey, R., Gaca, C. & VanderSalm, T. (2001) The use of smaller more flexible chest drains following open heart surgery: an initial evaluation. *Chest* **119**(1): 19–24.

Lazar, H., Hudson, H., McCann, J. *et al.* (1995) Gastrointestinal complications following cardiac surgery. *Cardiovascular Surgery* **3**(3): 341–4.

Leach, R.M. & Treacher, D.F. (2002) The pulmonary physician in critical care 2. Oxygen delivery and consumption in the critically ill. *Thorax* **57**(2): 170–77.

Leme, G., Canessa, R. & Urzua, J. (1998) Renal preservation in cardiac surgery. *Current Opinions in Anaesthesiology* **11**(1): 9–13.

Lim-Levy, F., Babler, S.A., Ge Groot-Kosolcharoen, J., Kosolcharoen, P. & Kroncke, G.M. (1986) Is milking and stripping chest tubes really necessary? *Annals of Thoracic Surgery* **42**: 77–80.

Loop, F.D., Lytle, B.W., Cosgrove, D.M. *et al.* (1990) Sternal wound complications after isolated coronary bypass grafting: early and late mortality, morbidity and cost of care. *Annals of Thoracic Surgery* **49**: 179–87.

Maglish, B., Schwartz, J. & Matheny, R. (1999) Outcomes improvement following minimally invasive direct coronary artery bypass surgery. *Critical Care Nursing Clinics of North America* **11**(2): 177–88.

Mahamid, E. (2000) Noninvasive positive-pressure ventilation in acute respiratory failure. *Care of the Critically Ill* **16**(2): 55–8.

Mahon, S.V., Berry, P.D., Jackson, M., Russell, G.N. & Pennefather, S.H. (1999) Thoracic epidural infusions for postthoracotomy pain: a comparison of fentanyl–bupivacaine mixtures vs fentanyl alone. *Anaesthesia* **54**(7): 641–6.

Matte, P., Jacquet, L., Van Dyck, M. & Goenen, M. (2000) Effects of conventional physiotherapy, continuous positive airway pressure and non-invasive ventilatory support with bi-level positive airway pressure after coronary artery bypass grafting. *Acta Anaesthesiologica Scandinavica* **44**: 75–81.

McCaughey, W. & Graham, J.L. (1982) The respiratory depression of epidural morphine: time course and effect of posture. *Anaesthesia* **37**: 990–95.

Mehta, S., Jay, G.D., Woolard, R.H. *et al.* (1997) Randomised continuous positive airway pressure in acute pulmonary oedema. *Critical Care Medicine* **25**: 620–28.

Melzack, R. & Wall, P.D. (1965) Pain mechanism: a new theory. *Science* **150**: 971–9.

Mermel, L.A. (2000) Prevention of intravascular catheter related infections. *Annals of Internal Medicine* **132**: 391–402.

Merskey, H. & Bogduk, N. (1994) *Classification of Chronic Pain: Descriptions of Chronic Pain Syndromes and Definition of Pain Terms. Report by the International Association for the Study of Pain Task Force on Taxonomy*, 2nd edn. IASP Press, Seattle.

Miller, K.M. & Perry, P.A. (1990) Relaxation technique and postoperative pain in patients undergoing cardiac surgery. *Heart and Lung* **19**: 136–46.

Mitch, W.E., Medina, R., Grieber, S. *et al.* (1994) Metabolic acidosis stimulates muscle protein degradation by activating the adenosine triphosphate-dependent pathway involving ubiquitin and proteasomes. *Journal of Clinical Investigations* **93**: 2127–33.

Moore, K. (1999) Cell biology of chronic wounds: the role of inflammation. *Journal of Wound Care* **8**: 345–8.

Morris, D. & St Claire, D. (1999) Management of patients following cardiac surgery. *Current Problems in Cardiology* **24**(4): 165–228.

Munnell, E.R. (1997) Thoracic drainage. *Annals of Thoracic Medicine* **63**: 1497–1502.

Murphy, D.F., Graziotti, P., Chalkiadis, G. & McKenna, M. (1994) Patient controlled analgesia: a comparison with nurse controlled intravenous opioid infusions. *Anaesthesia and Intensive Care* **2295**: 589–92.

Myles, P.S., Buckland, M.R., Cannon, G.B. *et al.* (1994) Comparison of patient controlled analgesia and nurse controlled analgesia after cardiac surgery. *Anaesthesia and Intensive Care* **22**(6): 672–8.

Newman, M., Kirchnere, J., Phillips-Bute, B. *et al.* (2001) Longitudinal assessment of neurocognitive function after coronary artery bypass graft. *New England Journal of Medicine* **344**: 395–402.

Niv, D. & Devor, M. (1998) Transition from acute to chronic pain. In: Aronoff, G.M. (ed.) *Evaluation and Treatment of Chronic Pain*, 3rd edn. Williams & Wilkins, Baltimore.

O'Brien, J. (1995) Developing and implementing a self learning packet on epidural analgesia. *Medical Surgical Nursing Journal* **4**(6): 438–44.

O'Halloran, P. & Brown, R. (1997) Patient controlled analgesia compared with nurse con-trolled infusion analgesia after heart surgery. *Intensive and Critical Care Nursing* **13**: 126–9.

Orchard, C.H. & Kentish, J.C. (1990) Effects of changes of pH on the contractile function of cardiac muscle. *American Journal of Physiology* **258**: C967–C981.

Orfanos, P., Ellis, E.R. & Johnstone, C. (1999) Effects of deep breathing exercises and ambulation on pattern of ventilation in postoperative patients. *Australian Journal of Physiotherapy* **45**: 173–82.

Owen, S. & Gould, D.J. (1997) Underwater seal chest drains: the patient's experience. *Journal of Clinical Nursing* **6**: 215–25.

Parkin, C. (2002) A retrospective audit of chest drain practice in a specialist cardiothoracic centre and concurrent review of chest drain literature. *Nursing in Critical Care* **7**(1): 30–36.

Perttunen, K., Tasmuth, T. & Kalso, E. (1999) Chronic pain after thoracic surgery: a follow up study. *Acta Anaesthesiologica Scandinavica* **43**: 563–7.

Peters, J. (1998) A review of the factors influencing non-recurrence of venous leg ulcers. *Journal of Clinical Nursing* **7**(1): 3–9.

Pierce, J.D., Piazza, D. & Naftel, D.C. (1991) Effects of two chest tube clearance protocols on drainage inpatients after myocardial revascularisation surgery. *Heart and Lung* **20**: 125–30.

Plowman, R. (1999) *The Socio-economic Burden of Hospital-acquired Infection*. Public Health Laboratory Service, London.

Pryor, J.A. & Webber, B.A. (2002) Physiotherapy techniques. In: Pryor, J.A. & Prasad, S.A. (eds) *Physiotherapy for Respiratory and Cardiac Problems: Adults and Paediatrics*, 3rd edn. Elsevier Science, London.

Puntillo, K. & Weiss, S.J. (1994) Pain: its mediators and associated morbidity in critically ill cardiovascular surgical patients. *Nursing Research* **43**: 31–5.

Rady, M., Ryan, T. & Starr, N. (1997) Early onset of acute pulmonary dysfunction after cardiovascular surgery: risk factors and clinical outcome. *Critical Care Medicine* **25**(11): 1831–9.

Rai, M. & Dexter, T. (2001) Intravascular catheters and sepsis. *Care of the Critically Ill* **17**(1): 21–5.

Ralley, F.E., Wynands, J.E., Ramasa, J.G. *et al.* (1988) The effects of shivering on oxygen consumption and carbon dioxide production in patients rewarming from hypothermic cardiopulmonary bypass. *Canadian Journal of Anaesthesia* **35**: 332–7.

Randolph, A.G., Cook, D.J., Gonzales, C.A. & Andrew, M. (1998) Benefit of heparin in central venous and pulmonary artery catheters: a meta-analysis of randomised con-trolled studies. *Chest* **113**: 165–71.

Ranganathan, J. (1989) Life in the fast track. *Health Service Journal* **99**(5179): 1468–9.

Reyes, A., Vega, G., Blancas, R., Morato, B., Moreno, J., Torrecilla, C. & Cereijo, E. (1997) Early vs conventional extubation after cardiac surgery with cardiopulmonary bypass. *Chest* **112**(1): 193–201.

Rho, R., Bridges, C. & Kocovic, D. (2000) Management of postoperative arrhythmias. *Seminars in Thoracic and Cardiovascular Surgery* **12**(4): 349–61.

Richards, K., Gibson, R. & Overton-McCoy, A.L. (2000) Effects of massage in acute and critical care. *American Association of Critical Care Nurses* **11**(1): 77–96.

Richardson, J., Sabanathan, S., Jones, J. *et al.* (1999a) A prospective, randomised comparison of preoperative and continuous balanced epidural or paravertebral bupivacaine on post thoracotomy pain, pulmonary function and stress responses. *British Journal of Anaesthesia* **83**: 387–92.

Richardson, J., Sabanathan, S. & Shah, R. (1999b) Post-thoracotomy spirometric lung function: the effect of analgesia. *Journal of Cardiovascular Surgery* **40**: 445–56.

Richardson, J. (2001) Postoperative epidural analgesia: introducing evidence based guidelines through an education and assessment process. *Journal of Clinical Nursing* **10**(2): 238–45.

Riley. J. (1995) Fast track cardiac care. *Nursing Standard* **9**(49): 55–6.

Riley, J. (2002) The ECG: principles and practice. In: Hatchett, R. & Thompson, D. (eds) *Cardiac Nursing: A Comprehensive Guide.* Churchill Livingstone, Edinburgh.

Rolstad, B.S., Ovington, L.G. & Harris, A. (2000) *Principles of Wound Management.* Mosby, London.

Rooney, P. (1995) Intravenous therapy. *Surgical Nurse* **8**(3): 4–8.

Rosenbaum, G., Klein, N. & Cinha, B. (1990) Poststernotomy mediastinitis. *Heart and Lung* **19**(4) 371–2.

Rosenthal, M.H. (1999) Intraoperative fluid management – what and how much? *Chest* **115**(5): 106S–112S.

Royston, D., Minty, B.D., Higenbottam, T.W. *et al.* (1985) The effect of surgery with cardiopulmonary bypass on alveolar–capillary barrier function in human beings. *Annals of Thoracic Surgery* **40**: 139–43.

Schaffer, M.R. & Barbul, A. (1996) Chemotherapy and wound healing. In: Lefor, A.T. (ed.) *Surgical Problems Affecting the Patient with Cancer.* Lippincott-Raven, Philadelphia.

Schierhout, G. & Roberts, I. (1998) Fluid resuscitation with colloid or crystalloid solutions in critically ill patients: a systematic review of randomised trials. *British Medical Journal* **316**: 961–4.

Scurr, J . (1988) Deep vein thrombosis: a continuing problem. *British Medical Journal* **297**: 28.

Seers, K. & Carroll, D. (1998) Relaxation techniques for acute pain management: a systematic review. *Journal of Advanced Nursing* **27**(3): 466–75.

Shapiro, B.A., Kacmarek, R.M., Cane, R.D. *et al.* (1991) *Clinical Application of Respiratory Care,* 4th edn. Mosby–Year Book Medical Publishers, Chicago.

Shirreffs, J. (1996) It's time to consider the alternative – even the controversial ones. *Journal of Health Education* **27**: 119–21.

Simonds, A.K. (2001) NIPPV in acute respiratory failure due to non-COPD disorders. In: Simonds, A.K. (ed.) *Non-invasive Respiratory Support: A Practical Handbook,* Edward Arnold, London.

Slaughter, T., Sreeram, G., Sharma, A., El-Moalem, H., East, C. & Greenberg, C. (2001) Reversible shear-mediated platelet dysfunction during cardiac surgery as assessed by the PFA-100® platelet function analyser. *Blood Coagulation and Fibrinolysis* **12**(2): 85–93.

Slinger, P.D. (1995) Perioperative fluid management for thoracic surgery: the puzzle of post pneumonectomy oedema. *Journal of Cardiothoracic and Vascular Anaesthesia* **9**: 442–51.

Smith, M.C.L. & Ellis, E.R. (2000) Is retained mucus a risk for the development of postoperative atelectasis and pneumonia? Implications for the physiotherapist. *Physiotherapy Theory and Practice* **16**: 69–80.

Sofer, D., Gurevitch, J., Shapira, I. *et al.* (1999) Sternal wound infections in patients after coronary artery bypass grafting using bilateral skeletonised internal mammary arteries. *Annals of Surgery* **229**(4): 585–90.

Soifer, N.E., Borzak, S., Edlin, B.R. & Weinstein, R.A. (1998) Prevention of peripheral venous complications with an intravenous therapy team: a randomised controlled study. *Archives of Internal Medicine* **158**: 473–7.

Stahle, E., Tammelin, A., Bergstrom, R., Hambreus, A., Nystrom, S.O. & Hansson, H.E. (1997) Sternal wound complications – incidence, microbiology and risk factors. *European Journal of Cardiothoracic Surgery* **11**: 1146–53.

Stamou, S., Dangas, G., Hill, P. *et al.* (2000) Atrial fibrillation after beating heart surgery. *American Journal of Cardiology* **86**(1): 64–7.

Stevenson, C.J. (1994) The psychophysiological effects of aromatherapy massage following cardiac surgery. *Complementary Therapies in Medicine* **2**(1): 27–35.

Stiller, K., Montarello, J., Wallace, M. *et al.* (1994) Efficacy of breathing and coughing exercises in the prevention of pulmonary complications after coronary artery surgery. *Chest* **105**: 741–7.

Taggart, D. (2002) Bilateral internal mammary artery grafting: are BIMA better? *Heart* **88**: 7–9.

Taggart, D.P., El-Fiky, M., Carter, R. *et al.* (1993) Respiratory dysfunction after uncomplicated cardiopulmonary bypass. *Annals of Thoracic Surgery* **56**: 1123–8.

Topf, M. & Thompson, S. (2001) Interactive relationships between hospital patients' noise induced stress and other stress with sleep. *Heart and Lung* **30**(4): 237–43.

Toto, K.H. (1998) Fluid balance assessment: the total perspective. *Critical Care Nursing Clinics of North America* **10**(4): 383–400.

Turfrey, D., Roy, D., Sutcliffe, N., Ramayya, P., Kenny, G. & Scott, N. (1997) Thoracic epidural anesthesia for CABG surgery: effects on post-operative complications. *Anaesthesia* **52**(11): 1090–95.

Turk, D.C. & Okifuji, A. (1999) Pain: assessment of patients' reporting of pain – an integrated perspective. *Lancet* **353**: 1784–8.

Utley, J.R., Thomason, M.E., Wallace, D.J. *et al.* (1989) Preoperative correlates of impaired wound healing after saphenous vein excision. *Journal of Thoracic Cardiovascular Surgery* **89**: 147–9.

Vaska, P. (1993) Sternal wound infections. *AACN Clinical Issues in Critical Care Nursing* **4**(3): 475–83.

Velanovich, V. (1989) Crystalloid versus colloid fluid resuscitation: a meta-analysis of mortality. *Surgery* **105**: 65–71.

Wait, J. (1996) Preoperative pulmonary evaluation. *Current Pulmonary and Critical Care Medicine* **17**: 252–4.

Wall, P.D. & Woolf, C.J. (1986) The brief and prolonged facilitatory effects of unmyelinated afferent input on the rat spinal cord are influenced by peripheral nerve section. *Neuroscience* **17**: 1199–1205.

Weiner, P., Man, A., Weiner, M. *et al.* (1997) The effect of incentive spirometry and inspiratory muscle training on pulmonary function after lung resection. *Journal of Thoracic and Cardiovascular Surgery* **113**: 552–7.

West, J.B. (2000) *Respiratory Physiology: The Essentials.* Lippincott/Williams & Wilkins, London.

Whaley, L. & Wong, D. (1989) *Essentials of Paediatric Nursing*, 3rd edn. Mosby, St Louis, MO.

Whitby, D.J. (1995) The biology of wound healing. *Surgery* 25–8.

White, J.M. (1999) Effects of relaxing music on cardiac autonomic balance and anxiety after acute myocardial infarction. *American Journal of Critical Care* **8**: 220–30.

Whitney, J.D. & Heitkemper, M.M. (1999) Modifying perfusion, nutrition and stress to promote wound healing in patients with acute wounds. *Heart and Lung* **28**(2): 123–33.

Yeager, M.P., Glass, D.D., Neff, R.K. & Brinck-Johnsen, T. (1987) Epidural anaesthesia and analgesia in high risk surgical patients. *Anaesthesiology* **66**: 729.

Zacharias, A. & Habib, R.H. (1996) Factors predisposing to median sternotomy complications: deep vs superficial infection. *Chest* **110**: 1173–8.

Further reading

Dealey, C. (1999) *The Care of Wounds: A Guide for Nurses*, Blackwell Science, London.

Pryor, J.A. & Prasad, S.A. (2002) *Physiotherapy for Respiratory and Cardiac Problems: Adults and Paediatrics*, 3rd edn. Churchill Livingstone, London.

Simonds, A.K. (ed.) (2001) *Non-invasive Respiratory Support: A Practical Handbook*. Edward Arnold, London.

Appendix: Post-operative assessment issues following cardiac surgery

Data	Method	Rationale	Possible action
Cardiac output	■ Central temperature	Hypothermia acts as a myocardial depressant	Actively warm with bair hugger, eliminate shivering, avoid administration of cold fluids
	■ Peripheral temperature, capillary refill, warmth and colour		
	■ Blood pressure	See below	
	■ Cardiac output monitoring, echocardiography	Useful to exclude causes of low cardiac output; cardiac tamponade and cardiac function	Titrate fluid and drug therapy against cardiac output recordings
Blood pressure	■ Arterial line	Arterial line more accurately reflects arterial pressure in the presence of low cardiac output or peripheral vasoconstriction	Gentle rewarming with blood/fluid titration and low-dose nitrates
		During rewarming, blood pressure is frequently labile	
	■ Guideline MAP <70 mmHg	MAP – reflects the pressure perfusing body organs	Maintain MAP with inotropes if necessary
	■ Systolic <120 mmHg	High systolic pressure increases the risk of bleeding from suture lines and increases afterload	Nitrates may successfully maintain systolic pressure <120 mmHg
Fluid balance	■ Guideline RAP 8–12 mmHg	Maintain filling pressure to those found optimal intra-operatively	Titrate fluid to maintain filling pressures: 6% Hetastarch/blood – see blood clotting section below
	■ LAP 12 mmHg		
	■ Maintain urine output >0.5 ml/kg body weight	Initial large diuresis resulting from CPB should reduce within 2 hours	Administer frusemimde to maintain urine output

Blood loss	■ Chest drains positioned in mediastinum and pleura ■ Observe blood drainage, clot formation within tubing ■ Suction pressure −5 kPa (30–40 cm H₂O)	Excessive bleeding may lead to hypovolaemia while decreased bleeding or clot formation may inhibit drainage and result in cardiac tamponade Guidelines <4–5 ml/kg in the first 3–4 hours Pressure should maintain a slow consistent bubbling	Facilitate drainage by 45 degree head-up position See blood clotting below Exploration of surgical site may be necessary
ECG	■ Continuous ECG to monitor heart rate and rhythm	Observe arrhythmias – particularly PVCs Maintain heart rate 80–100 bpm	Treat arrhythmias that lead to cardiovascular compromise Use nitrates, oxygen and reduce myocardial oxygen demand Maintain heart rate with pharmacological agents such as isoprenaline or epicardial pacing
	■ 12 lead ECG to monitor ischaemia or MI (R wave progression, new LBBB, Q wave development)	Ischaemia may indicate coronary vein graft spasm or myocardial oxygen supply/demand imbalance. MI may occur intra-operatively CKMB and troponin I are raised following cardiac surgery	Administer oxygen and nitrates to maximise myocardial oxygen supply while reducing shivering, work of breathing, pain and anxiety
Electrolytes	■ Serum electrolytes on return from surgery and daily thereafter	Actively manage potassium to reduce risk of arrhythmias Low potassium may result from stress response or profound diuresis Hyperkalaemia may result from cardioplegic solutions, renal dysfunction	IV potassium supplements. Large doses of IV potassium should be administered through a central line
	■ Maintain serum K⁺ 4.5–5.0 mmol/l ■ Maintain serum magnesium 1.4–2.2 mmol/l	Magnesium mimics potassium in the effect upon the heart Hypomagnesaemia may result from diuretics	Administer IV magnesium to improve stroke volume and reduce arrhythmias

Contd

Appendix: *Contd*

Data	Method	Rationale	Possible action
Blood clotting	■ Monitor haematocrit ■ Maintain >25% ■ Aim for Hb >8 g/dl ■ ACT <160	Reduce risk of bleeding and low blood pressure Adequate haemoglobin is necessary for good oxygenation	Use blood to maintain Hb >8 g/dl Stop pre-operative anti-platelets (aspirin/clopidogrel) 1 week prior to surgery. Stop warfarin 3 days before
Respiratory status	■ Arterial blood gases ■ Aim for PO_2 >10 kPa PCO_2 <7 kPa SaO_2 >95% BE +/−3 ■ Chest X-ray	Maintain adequate oxygenation and CO_2 removal Acidosis depresses cardiac function Check position of lines and chest tubes and for presence of pleural effusions/ haemothorax or atelectasis	Extubate as soon as possible. Administer oxygen via face mask to maintain adequate oxygenation
Blood glucose	■ Record blood glucose 4 hourly	Catecholamines raise blood glucose Insulin secretion is decreased on CPB or with hypothermia and there is a blunted response to insulin for 24 hours following CPB	Sliding scale insulin if diabetic to <10 mmol <15 mmol/l in non-diabetic
Neurology	■ Neurological assessment	Severe agitation on waking may indicate neurological deficit	Re-sedate for 12 hours and re-assess
Pain relief	■ Regular pain assessment with pain scale ■ Heart rate/respiratory rate ■ Blood pressure ■ Non-verbal expression/agitation	Inadequate pain relief limits respiratory effort and mobilisation hence predisposes to chest infections Excessive use of opiates causes respiratory depression Patient-controlled analgesia avoids subjective interpretation of pain	PCA/bolus dose – morphine NSAIDs may lead to renal impairment Epidural analgesis following cardiac surgery is problematical with increased risk of spinal haematoma Support sternal wound during coughing or moving

7
Returning Home

The longer-term success of surgery, measured in terms of quality of life, will depend not only on the expertise of the cardiothoracic team during the perioperative period, but also on preparation for discharge and ongoing support once at home. The trend towards even shorter periods of hospitalisation for surgery continues, and innovative models of care, to both prepare patients for surgery and to support them in the post-operative period and beyond, are required so that any physical, psychological, social and financial consequences are minimised. The period of hospitalisation for surgery focuses very much on the acute aspect of care but additional models are required if the patient and carer are to be prepared effectively for the return home.

This chapter explores the difficulties that patients might face once discharged home. In the pre-admission chapter (Chapter 4) a framework was offered to help the nurse carry out a psychosocial assessment. This framework is just as appropriate when preparing the patient for discharge, and using the four dimensions – pathophysiological (symptoms), cognitive, behavioural and social factors – will facilitate exploration of key issues in this section. Information-giving alone prior to discharge is unlikely to lead to successful adjustment following surgery. Opportunities need to be made available so that patients can develop the confidence, knowledge and skills to cope more effectively, thereby gaining greater control and independence with improved quality of life. An overview of theoretical and philosophical issues underpinning such approaches will contribute towards increasing the effectiveness of the nurse's role in this area.

Earlier discharge

Traditionally, the hospital length of stay following cardiac surgery was 10 days, but this has fallen progressively, first to 7 then 5 over the past decade (Riegal *et al.* 1996; Dunstan and Riddle 1997). This trend, while due mainly to changes in perioperative management (Maglish *et al.* 1999), has also been influenced by the need for cost containment. Even following thoracic surgery involving resection there has been a move towards earlier discharge, so that, generally, cardiothoracic patients may be discharged home 3–4 days after major surgery. These relatively recent developments are still uncharted waters as there are many questions unanswered regarding the long-term implications of early discharge.

With more women presenting for surgery, more elderly (often with comorbidity), more ethnic minority groups and patients requiring 'redo' procedures, health care needs following discharge are increasingly complex. Following cardiac surgery, for example, there are striking differences between men and women, with the latter having worse health experiences. These differences are sustained one year after cardiac surgery and interventions need to be targeted to enhance recovery, reduce morbidity and improve quality of life (Jenkins & Gortner 1998).

Adverse psychological and physical functioning can be found as late as six months following cardiothoracic surgery (Moore 1995). A significant number of patients will suffer anxiety and depression, and although emotional reactions are to be expected these may cause further distress and disability if intense and prolonged. Mood is often fairly labile following major cardiothoracic surgery and the patient and carer may need reassurance and help in dealing with these emotions. Despite surgery, patients may still be frightened to resume their social contacts or return to work and may still have fears over the future (Jaarsma *et al.* 1995). There are likely to be differences between patients who have restorative surgery and those who need surgery for cancer. In one study of patients following cardiac surgery (*n* = 534), the Short Form 36 Health Survey (SF-36) showed an improvement in all eight dimensions at 6–12 months (Yun *et al.* 1999). In comparison, another study involving patients having undergone thoracic surgery (*n* = 123) showed that whereas pain and other physical constructs had improved after one month, mental health, role limitations secondary to mental health and health perception had not (Mangione *et al.* 1997).

Patient education

Caregivers as well as patients can experience a wide range of emotions and also need information related to the length of recovery, lifestyle modification, side-effects of medication and enhancing quality of life. Caregiver support is crucial in the post-operative period, but careful preparation is needed so that carers are not overwhelmed (Jickling & Graydon 1997). If inadequately informed and supported regarding lifestyle changes resulting from surgery, there may be increased anxiety for both patient and caregiver, with delayed recovery and increased readmission rates for the patient.

Initial patient education must involve instruction on what to expect regarding sensations, rate of recovery, skills to perform, symptoms to observe for and contact details for ongoing support. This will help patients to increase their understanding of how to manage the post-operative course and how to regain social, family and work roles and return to as active a life as possible. Knowledge and ability regarding any lifestyle changes should be enhanced, but common sense should be exercised regarding risk modification in each individual case.

It is important to remember that, for most patients undergoing cardiac and thoracic surgery, the procedure is not curative. For example, following thoracic surgery for lung cancer, a realistic plan needs to be devised so that healing is optimised but the regimen not so rigid that quality of life is sacrificed. An important objective following CABG will be risk factor modification to slow the evolution of further pathology that may threaten the coronary artery grafts. Cardiac surgery does not halt the process of atheroma development and 10% of saphenous vein grafts are occluded by the end of the first year and approximately 50% of coronary grafts are occluded after 10 years. Although grafts are threatened in the immediate post-operative period because of technical problems or thrombosis, there is accelerated atherosclerosis several months following surgery that threatens their long-term patency. Patients are therefore prescribed an antiplatelet, which they should start the day following surgery and continue for life. Although aspirin has been used successfully for many years, not all patients can tolerate the drug. An alternative antiplatelet agent is clopidogrel. However, this must be taken three times daily. Not surprisingly, complicated regimens are inversely related to compliance and are best avoided (Claxton *et al.* 2001). Continued attention to risk factor modification remains important.

Patients are often very worried about the risk of long-term disability associated with lung surgery (Cykert *et al.* 2000). Functional assessment of patients after health care interventions is becoming increasingly important and there is a need for a more comprehensive understanding of the effects of thoracic surgery on patients' functional and quality of life outcomes (Handy *et al.* 2002). Patients requiring resection for lung cancer are likely to have greater impairment of physical and emotional functioning with poorer psychosocial reserves pre-operatively and further problems in these areas following surgery. What is clear is that there is a discrepancy between what doctors consider important post-operatively (mortality and complications) and what the patient perceives as important (persistent physical disability) (Handy *et al.* 2002).

Symptom control

Problems experienced by patients following cardiothoracic surgery are often related to wounds, pain, fatigue, sleep disturbance and problems with dietary intake, and these can persist for up to eight weeks (Moore 1995).

The patient will understandably have concerns about the surgical wounds. In cardiac surgery there may be a sternal wound as well as a donor site where the graft was harvested. Following thoracic surgery there may be a posterolateral incision. Although surgical wounds may be smaller as a result of minimally invasive techniques, the principles are the same. A degree of redness, soreness and itching is to be expected during the healing process but excessive discharge, particularly where there is an unpleasant smell, should be reported. Wounds are best left uncovered and gently washed with water and non-perfumed soap and patted dry.

The nurse may need to take time in helping the patient to differentiate between different types of somatic pain. Chest discomfort following surgery is usual but the patient may misinterpret this as the return of their old problem, resulting in a great deal of worry and distress. Chest pain has been identified as the main variable negatively influencing return to work in cardiac patients (Speziale *et al.* 1996). Cardiac and thoracic surgery involves major procedures, which are often lengthy, and this taxes the reserves of most individuals, who often complain of varying degrees of musculo-skeletal discomfort and profound fatigue.

In the pre-operative period patients must be made aware of the changes to expect and that these may persist for some time. Instruction may involve helping to anticipate fatigue as well as strategies to promote adequate rest and sleep. Heavy work, particularly involving strain at the wound site, should be avoided, although increasing graded exercise is to be encouraged.

In surgery for cancer the best that the patient can hope for is removal of as much of the tumour as possible, but for many, some degree of pathology will remain, possibly contributing to fatigue. The ongoing fatigue experienced by patients is often a reminder of the ongoing battle being waged against the cancer, and for those unaware of their diagnosis this can lead to further distress and frustration. Fatigue can be all-consuming and permeate all aspects of the patient's existence. Wendy Harpham, a doctor who developed non-Hodgkin's lymphoma and has first-hand experience of the frustration of fatigue following cancer therapy, offers a deeply personal and valuable insight into the difficulties faced by individuals (Harpham 1999). She refers to 'Post-cancer Fatigue' for the fatigue that persists when treatment has ended, and argues that the introduction of this additional terminology for talking about the fatigue that accompanies serious or chronic illnesses may facilitate healing communication between patients and their health care teams and/or with families, friends and co-workers.

> More often there is a mismatch between inner and outer life . . . Survivors often look better to others than they feel. When patients [with cancer] are bald or walking on crutches, everyone expects them to have limits. When incisions are healed and hair has grown back, however, friends and family shower tired survivors with compliments about how healthy they look, even how energetic they appear (or sound over the phone) Survivors' attempts to explain their fatigue are often greeted with assurances, 'Well, you look great!' (Harpham 1999: 183)

Patients who have undergone resection for cancer will need careful follow-up and the specialist nurse has an important role here. Even when medical treatment is optimised, problems may still be experienced and the nurse should be knowledgeable about other resources available when referral is necessary. When all other avenues seem to have been exhausted, complementary therapy may be of benefit.

Exploring cognitions

We ignore the patient's cognitions at our peril and time should be taken to explore the patient's concerns and understanding regarding, for example, causation, treatment expectations and perceived susceptibility/vulnerability. Cognitions both fuel our emotions and help determine our behavioural responses. Diary-keeping by the patient provides a record of problems experienced, including frequency and severity as well as precipitating, exacerbating and alleviating factors. Recent episodes can be explored in detail to examine associated cognitions, behaviours and physiological symptoms. This will help the nurse in offering possible alternative explanations and help both to identify areas to be targeted in action plans and to ensure development of more appropriate strategies.

Motivational interviewing

Exploring cognitions is particularly important in attempting any risk modification in patients and any lifestyle change cannot be brought about by information alone. Motivating patients to change their behaviour involves the nurse increasing the patient's awareness of the need to change, identifying how to make any changes and then offering suggestions to maintain this state. Motivational interviewing is a technique combining both humanistic and behavioural principles and the model of the change cycle by Prochaska and DiClemente (1984) outlined in Fig. 7.1 offers a useful framework for this approach. The model has been used widely in smoking cessation, exercise and other health behaviour.

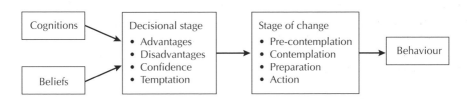

Fig. 7.1 Stages of change model.

The stages identified in Fig. 7.1 do not always occur in order, nor is there a predetermined time frame for any change. It is also important to realise that although someone may have been diagnosed with cardiac or respiratory disease and perhaps even undergone surgery, they may not be ready to undertake lifestyle changes. Even in the post-operative period, patients may not have reached the contemplation stage. Conversely, patients may be shocked by the urgency of surgery and motivated and committed to making changes to their lifestyle, such as giving up smoking. Indeed, this action stage may have been reached before surgery. However, it cannot be assumed that the maintenance stage will be sustained and movement in either direction is possible in the change cycle.

Social learning theory

Another theoretical approach to behavioural change that addresses cognitive processes is that of social learning theory. Described by Bandura (1977), this theory has been widely applied to health behaviours and again emphasises the interplay of cognitions, behaviour and the environment (Fig. 7.2). It suggests that behaviour change is more likely if there is belief and confidence in one's ability to perform the behaviour. This belief, known as self-efficacy, can be influenced by persuasion from others in social or professional groups, observation and modelling as well as by the successful performance of a behaviour, which offers positive feedback and physiological feedback. Social learning theory suggests that behaviours can be both learned or unlearned. Therefore learning through modelling behaviours is an important component of this theory.

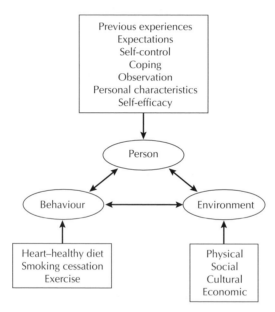

Fig. 7.2 Factors influencing behaviour, utilising social learning theory.

A patient who has low self-esteem is likely to have lower expectations of their abilities to modify their behaviours and may be influenced more by environmental conditions that may either facilitate or inhibit the change. For example, a person with low levels of self-efficacy may not believe they can climb the stairs following cardiothoracic surgery without getting breathless and so prefer to stay downstairs. Someone with greater self-efficacy, on the other hand, is more likely to believe they can perform the necessary skills.

Confidence can be increased through various strategies: observing others, persuasion and previous experience, and the cardiothoracic surgical nurse can use these to facilitate the patient's post-operative behaviours. Studies show that recovery is enhanced and distress alleviated when patients who have similar illnesses and who are facing similar procedures are placed together in shared rooms during the period of hospitalisation (Kulik *et al.* 1996). This not only assists with the crisis of surgery but also helps prepare the patient for the process of recovery. It is likely that during such times, similar others are able to offer standards for emotional and behavioural self-evaluation and may also be a source of information, coping assistance and role modelling (Helgeson & Taylor 1993).

Theory of reasoned action

The theory of reasoned action (Ajzen & Fishbein 1980) has also been widely used to predict health behaviours. Underlying this theory is the concept that behaviour is related to beliefs and intention (Fig. 7.3). Influencing beliefs are the perceptions of those that we value – spouses, friends, health care professionals. For many young people, stopping smoking or drinking may involve losing credibility with friends, perceived as a more powerful reason for continuing than the health gains from quitting.

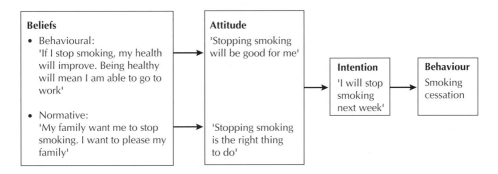

Fig. 7.3   Theory of reasoned action applied to smoking cessation.

Continuing patient education

In addition to using social cognition models the principles of patient education referred to in Chapter 4 must continue to be utilised. Awareness of the factors which facilitate adult learning will contribute towards increased effectiveness of patient education strategies and it is useful to remember the following:

- Adults' readiness to learn is influenced by awareness of a problem or a major life event
- Adults prefer to be self-directed
- They want to participate actively in their learning
- They have past experiences that impact upon learning and can be used as a learning resource
- They learn by problem solving
- They value information seen as relevant and immediately applicable

Repetition will help to reinforce information given and the use of multimedia is also likely to enhance both individual and group sessions.

Facilitating adaptive behavioural responses

There are a number of behavioural responses that the nurse needs to be aware of and, as identified in Chapter 4, these can be classified as those that are health promoting and those that are potentially health damaging. Health-promoting behaviours may involve the patient and carer in learning skills that enable them to cope with wounds, wound drains (e.g. empyema), drug regimens and so on. The period before discharge will also offer an opportunity to reinforce self-management skills in those patients who have co-morbidity such as asthma or COPD where effectiveness of inhaler technique and peak flow recording can be checked.

Health-promoting behaviours will also involve lifestyle modification possibly related to diet, smoking and exercise, with any advice and suggested routines individualised. It should be remembered that a major component of a person's perceived independence is the ability to carry out the activities of daily living. This is where nursing models can be useful in helping the nurse to identify where possible deficits exist. Functional ability in the first two weeks following surgery may be well below the pre-operative status and increase anxiety during this time (Rudeker & Brassard 1996). Strategies to encourage activity and gain confidence may assist both the patient and their family through the forthcoming weeks.

Referral to an occupational therapist may be necessary. This will ensure that everything possible is done to promote self-caring, which, for a small number of patients, may require a home assessment.

Physiotherapists and nursing staff actively encourage daily exercise by walking with the patient in hospital and assisting them climb stairs from day 3 onwards. Levels of exercise can be encouraged in the hospital environment by the ward layout – walking to the day room or bathroom is frequently longer than the walks around a house at home. With ever shorter lengths of hospital stay, exercise regimens are likely to become an important issue that must be addressed by home care programmes. Patients should therefore be discharged home with an exercise programme that indicates incremental increases in intensity. This will then guide the patient and can be reinforced by the nurse at each home visit (Penque *et al.* 1999).

Behaviours which are health compromising may be indicative of poor coping and may not be evident at the time of discharge. Assessment on follow-up visits should involve exploration of this area with both patients and carer. Where difficulties are being experienced, the nurse will need to check on symptom control, cognitions and social support. Where behavioural responses are maladaptive, increasing distress for both patient and carer, referral to a counsellor or cognitive behavioural therapist may be necessary.

Social support

Social support has been associated with decreased cardiac mortality, better physical and psychological status of cardiac patients and their caregivers, and better adherence to treatment regimens (Moser 1994). In most chronic illness groups, social support is a crucial factor in helping patients to cope. It is not known exactly how social support contributes to health status but emotional support, esteem support, sense of belonging, instrumental support and informational support are all likely to have cognitive effects by improving self-esteem and perhaps behavioural effects by making it easier to adopt healthier lifestyles (Amick & Ockene 1994).

Historically, much external support was perceived to come from a spouse providing both emotional and tangible support. Indeed, early work on recovery from cardiovascular disease has demonstrated improved outcome and reduced mortality and morbidity following a myocardial infarction in those patients that were married (Moser 1994), while others have suggested that social support may be an important factor in preventing coronary heart disease (Tilden & Weinert 1987; Riegal 1989). However, the nature of the support offered by the spouse was not investigated until more recently. Similarly, social networks were assumed to provide positive forms of support without any prior evaluation of the nature of networks. Some relationships within networks, however, may not provide support but indeed act as a stressor. For example, a large social network may leave the recipient with a feeling of indebtedness that could provide a negative element and be counterproductive. Social relationships are changing and we can no longer think in terms of the traditional family. More research is needed into the role of social support and how this can be enhanced across a wide range of diverse family units.

Support groups have been used to provide an external mechanism of support for people with a chronic illness and may be associated with national organisations such as the British Cardiac Patients Association and Breathe Easy (British Lung Foundation). Through national or regional meetings they may offer support in the form of education, learning from others and possibly even teaching those undergoing similar experiences. Although assumed to have a positive effect upon adjustment to a chronic illness or recovery, the evidence is scarce.

Effective performance of various social roles is important in shaping our self-concept and self-esteem outlined earlier in this chapter. Difficulties with symptoms, changing self-concept and poor communication between partners may lead to problems with intimacy following surgery. Yet loss of intimacy within a relationship can further erode the patient's former self-concept, resulting in feelings of poor self-worth with low self-esteem (Margereson 2001).

Sexual dysfunction is not uncommon in someone with cardiovascular disease, possibly caused by medication (such as beta blockers), fear and anxiety, in either the patient or their partner. Yet the risk of an adverse cardiac event is low, with the risk of triggering a myocardial infarction in patients with a history of coronary heart disease of 2.9%. This is not significantly higher than in those with no history of the disease (2.5%) (Muller *et al.* 1996). Elsewhere it has been suggested that sexual activity with one's normal partner is no more stressful to the heart than many other activities such as walking one mile or climbing a flight of stairs (Tardif 1989; Jackson *et al.* 1999). Therefore, following successful surgical revacularisation, patients should be encouraged to resume previous sexual activity. In addition, when encouraged to take regular exercise, this small risk may be reduced still further to equate with those without a diagnosis of coronary heart disease (Muller *et al.* 1996). It is therefore useful to counsel patients and their families regarding resumption of normal sexual relationships. Although Sildenafil (Viagra™) is now available to help men with erectile dysfunction, this cannot be used alongside nitrate therapy or in patients with low blood pressure.

Expressing sexuality is an important activity of daily living, and following cardiothoracic surgery the nurse should reassure the patient and partner that any sexual concerns are legitimate. Sexual issues are often ignored in health care encounters but should be explored just like any other activity of daily living. Neither should it be assumed that only married patients have such concerns. Intimacy in a close relationship is important to all, including the elderly, those in a partnership and those living alone as well as those with chronic illness/disability. Addressing sexual issues post-operatively may simply involve giving information about the effects of surgery and medication on sexuality, together with general guidance on sexual health. Other issues to be addressed may include conserving energy, controlling physical symptoms, the importance of touch and communicating more openly with partners about sexual needs. Effective control of symptoms such as pain, dyspnoea, insomnia, fatigue and anaemia is important. Some problems of a physical nature may need to be addressed by the doctor.

Specialist nurses working in a cardiothoracic setting must ensure that they are able to offer appropriate guidance where patients are experiencing difficulty with intimacy, but where there are complex psychosocial factors involved then referral to specialist support may be needed

Support strategies

Hospital at home

One solution for managing the trend towards shorter and shorter hospital stays is 'hospital at home' schemes. In the current health care climate where hospitals are reserved for the very ill and there is ever increasing pressure on beds, we must look to alternative models of care to achieve the desired outcomes from surgery. Hospital at home models frequently rely upon care pathways and protocols. The care pathway will describe the typical course of treatment and should be designed by a multi-disciplinary team. This will ensure that the hospital at home scheme is not managed solely by the nursing staff but retains the multi-professional approach to care that would otherwise have been provided in the hospital. The use of a pathway also facilitates coordinated care by the practice nurse/district nurse/heath visitor. Some hospital at home schemes utilise hospital staff to provide an outreach service. Although this may ensure continuation between hospital care and the home it does not necessarily promote the continuation of care into the community. Adopting a similar shared care approach to that advocated during the wait for cardiac surgery may be an appropriate and more cost effective service.

An effective system of care will ensure that the person responsible for individualising the pathway has attended ward rounds and become familiar with the patient and their operative procedure. While in hospital, patients are frequently anxious and any detailed information regarding medications, exercising and chest physiotherapy may be more effective if undertaken once anxiety levels have decreased in the home care setting. Good glucose control in the diabetic patient is seen as increasingly important in delaying atheroma formation and therefore in delaying coronary graft occlusion, and patients may be discharged on insulin. When this is a new skill for the patient and their family, home support for education, reinforcement and supervision may be necessary.

When instituted carefully, home care can bridge the continuum of care between the inpatient phase and the community, and continue to assist recovery from surgery with attention to possible lifestyle changes. The costs of care may be higher than conventional hospital care with no significant differences in outcome (Penque *et al.* 1999). However, home care does leave a hospital bed free for another patient. How it shifts the scarce personnel resources is unclear and warrants further study.

Yet home care places a greater burden of responsibility upon the caregiver. Research related to the family experience with a chronic illness identifies four major ways in which the caregiver may impact upon the health of the patient. These include, the disease process itself, symptoms, degree of disability and the patient's emotional response (Kerns & Weiss 1994). Following surgery the family can remind the patient about medication, physical exercise and deep breathing regimens influencing recovery and assisting in symptom control. Providing support and encouragement to continue with social activities or return to work may include driving the person to work or on shopping trips. This is likely to impact favourably upon well-being and self-esteem, reduce anxiety and depression and contribute towards recovery. But for the carer the burden may be further increased as this commitment may involve significant investment in terms of emotion and time. Families, therefore, not only play an important part in the rehabilitation of the patient following cardiothoracic surgery, but are also affected themselves, possibly developing feelings of anger or depression. Before discharge home, it is therefore important to consider the home situation and, if necessary, to arrange for a period of convalescence. This should be assessed prior to hospital admission so that discharge planning can begin. Hospital discharge should not be delayed for social reasons.

Telephone support

Telephone calls following hospital discharge have been used without demonstrating any reduction in anxiety and depression (Roebuck 1999), although they may provide a 'feel-good factor' (Johnson 2000). Utilising technology to provide a more formal system of care may result in positive benefits to both reduce post-operative anxiety in the patient and their family and facilitate empowerment. One such model has been used in the USA for chronic disease management that may prove useful for the post-operative patient. 'Home talk', a disease management system, telephones the patient with pre-programmed questions and at scheduled times (Stricklin *et al.* 2000). The patient responds with a touch-tone reply and the nurse is notified of the results. Although this may be viewed as an impersonal service and open to error, it provides a service of home care that utilises current technology.

Another model of care is that of 'tele-home care'. Used widely for chronic disease management (Bowles & Danskey 2002), episodic care (Yerge-Cole 2001) and recovery from surgery (Brennan *et al*. 2001), it can assist early discharge. Here, booklets, tapes and videos can be used to provide information and reinforce skills such as breathing techniques or other behaviours. Self-monitoring of physiological parameters, such as oxygen saturation levels, blood pressure and ECG are facilitated and the data reported via a tele-link to health care staff. These staff can then advise the patient of any necessary alterations to their treatment and medication. Tele-home care enables patients to be self-directed and to actively participate in the recovery and rehabilitation process. It also enables the health care provider to reinforce information and to individualise and monitor regimens.

Not all patients following cardiac or thoracic surgery will complete a formal rehabilitation programme. Provision remains somewhat ad hoc, but where such a programme is available, it can contribute to the patient's recovery. The next section outlines the principles of rehabilitation.

Cardiac rehabilitation

Following cardiac surgery, angina may be abolished or significantly reduced yet quality of life frequently is disappointing. Many patients either fail to return to work or do so for only a few months. As the aim of cardiac rehabilitation includes the improvement of physical, social and psychological functioning (Thompson *et al*. 1996),it appears appropriate to consider the inclusion of the person following cardiac surgery into the growing number of cardiac rehabilitation programmes already developed to care for the person following myocardial infarction (MI). Indeed, the National Service Framework (DoH 2000) identifies the need for such programmes to widen their entry criteria to include those who have undergone cardiac surgery. Reported benefits of cardiac rehabilitation include enhanced physical fitness, increased confidence and improved health perception (Thompson & Lewin 2000), and a large meta-analysis of trials following MI demonstrated that cardiac rehabilitation significantly reduces cardiovascular mortality (O'Connor *et al*. 1989). However, the benefits for the person following cardiac surgery are less clear.

Evidence suggests that exercise improves graft patency and that an exercise programme should be commenced as soon as possible following surgery, possibly as early as the first two weeks (Nakai *et al*. 1987; Carrel & Mohacsi 1998). More recent work has demonstrated that although cardiac surgery improves myocardial ischaemia and functional capacity, when followed by a phase III cardiac rehabilitation programme 6–8 weeks following surgery, functional capacity improved only marginally (Ross *et al*. 2000; Sharma & McLeod 2001) or not at all (Wright *et al*. 2002). However, one important issue must be considered here. Cardiac rehabilitation services in the UK have mainly developed to meet the needs of patients following a MI and although providing this service at 6 weeks may be appropriate for this group, further work is necessary to determine the time at which rehabilitation following cardiac surgery provides maximum benefit.

Complete healing of the sternal wound following traditional cardiac surgery may not be complete until 6 weeks following surgery, and so certain precautions may be necessary for the person who starts earlier forms of exercise. Therefore, when encouraged in the early stages of recovery, exercises should avoid uncontrolled movements of the shoulders and arms, and swimming is best avoided until the wound is dry (Carrel & Mohacsi 1998). Where there is some degree of reduced left ventricular function, it is advisable to wait 3–6 weeks before commencing an exercise-based programme (AACPR 1999). In health, moderate exercise will increase heart rate and myocardial contractility (Skarvan 2000), whereas in ill health, moderate increases in heart rate may prove harmful.

The exercise effect

Exercise, both dynamic (isotonic) and static (isometric) has long been associated with cardiovascular benefit. As exercising muscles need more oxygen, the cardiac output increases (through increased heart rate and stroke volume) and the arteries of exercising skeletal muscle vasodilate. The heart rate increases through sympathetic nervous system activation, while changes in the stroke volume occur through increased skeletal muscle pump activity and constriction of the skeletal veins. Both these factors contribute towards an increased preload to the heart. Even when not competitive, exercise increases catecholamine release with both inotropic and chronotropic cardiac effects. Applying the principles of the Frank–Starling law (see Chapter 3, page 55), it is clear how, through alterations in both the preload and inotropic state, the exercising heart shifts the curve upwards and to the left and contributes towards an increase in cardiac output.

Dynamic exercise involves rhythmic contraction and relaxation of the muscles through activities such as walking or jogging. The systolic blood pressure is likely to rise while the diastolic pressure remains largely unchanged (Smith & Kampine 1990) or may even decrease slightly as the vasculature of the exercising muscles dilates. Exercise training that involves dynamic exercise increases the ventricular cavity size and so may provide cardiovascular benefit, and 20–30 minutes of exercise, three times per week may provide these benefits (Smith & Kampine 1990). This concurs with the current guidelines for exercise-based cardiac rehabilitation (DoH 2000). The National Service Framework for CHD suggests a period of 40 minutes which should include a warm-up and cool-down period either side of the exercise. Warm-up and cool-down are important. Dynamic exercise increases the activity of the skeletal pumping system and will increase venous return. It is therefore important that the heart rate is gradually slowed so that this increased venous return does not overload a failing heart.

In static exercise, such as resistance training, the muscles are maintained in a state of contraction, afterload is increased and the diastolic and systolic blood pressure may increase. Lifting a heavy shopping bag following cardiac surgery will invoke this same static exercise response, increasing the blood pressure, heart rate and consequently increasing myocardial oxygen demand. Following surgery, patients should therefore be advised to avoid lifting weights greater than 10 kg. If cardiac surgery follows a period of immobility, the muscles will have become deconditioned and lifting even 10 kg may be difficult. In such instances the weight lifted should be slowly increased. An important feature of cardiac rehabilitation is to restore the ability to perform previous social or work activities.

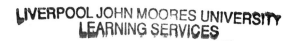

The trained heart is able to decrease diastolic pressure and so decrease myocardial oxygen demand and possibly reduce angina. Unfortunately these benefits are rapidly lost following a few weeks of inactivity. Rehabilitation therefore is useful to establish a pattern of exercise that affords cardiovascular benefit, an improved lipid profile and reduces blood pressure and weight while enhancing well-being.

Exercise issues for the diabetic patient

With the increasing number of people diagnosed with type II diabetes and the increased likelihood that they will have undergone revascularisation for CHD, specific attention to encouraging exercise in this population needs to be considered. Diabetic patients may have peripheral neuropathies and are at an increased risk of silent ischaemia. They may also have autonomic neuropathy and orthostatic hypotension. All these may influence the exercise regimen and patients should be advised to report any dizziness or excessive sweating at an early stage in their exercise, while staff should be vigilant to observe for early signs of myocardial ischaemia. Maintaining safety during bouts of exercise is particularly important, therefore. Both low and high blood sugar levels may also occur in response to exercise. Pre-exercise blood sugar levels of >7 mmol/l and <12.0 mmol/l should ensure safe exercise. Patients should also be advised to avoid exercising within two hours following a meal and, if using insulin, to inject into their abdomen rather than an exercising muscle.

CPB and cognitive dysfunction

Another consideration following cardiac surgery is the rehabilitation of someone who has some degree of cognitive dysfunction associated with cardiopulmonary bypass. An exercise-based rehabilitation programme has been shown to improve motor skills (Ng & Tam 2000) which may minimise any minor motor skills deficits encountered post-operatively. For the patient who has experienced a more profound neurological insult such as a cerebrovascular accident, more intense and prolonged rehabilitation to restore motor function will be required.

Encouraging attendance at cardiac rehabilitation

However, despite the proven benefit of cardiac rehabilitation following MI (Oldridge *et al.* 1992; Heller *et al.* 1993) poor attendance rates, particularly among women and ethnic minority groups, persist (Ades *et al.* 1992; Thomas *et al.* 1996). Increasingly it is recognised that regular attendance is less likely in the elderly, women, those in the lower socio-economic groups and in those living some distance away from the programme, and this has led to the development of home-based rehabilitation. Additionally this may be useful for those who return to work following their surgery and would prefer to undertake exercise in their own time. However, home-based rehabilitation does not offer the same benefits in terms of social support and networking and motivation may be reduced as a result.

Another factor that has been noted to reduce the uptake to cardiac rehabilitation following an MI is if the person has previously attended (Melville *et al.* 1999). Not all patients undergoing cardiac surgery will have experienced an MI, but for those that have, and who have previously attended cardiac rehabilitation, the focus of the programme must be stressed. It will enable them to revisit stress management, self-care behaviours and gain confidence in exercising thereby improving their chances of a successful outcome to the operation.

Increased hospital readmissions and outpatient or community services may offset any economic benefit gained by earlier discharge home (Lazar *et al.* 2001). However, following an effective cardiac rehabilitation programme the patient will have learnt skills to care for themselves and monitor their condition and so benefit from the reduced hospital stay.

It has become well established that women are less likely to attend cardiac rehabilitation, have greater negative emotions and less social support (Moore 1995). Women's exercise patterns also tail off following cardiac surgery and formal rehabilitation (Moore *et al.* 1998). This makes clear the need for an extended period of rehabilitation. Brennan *et al.* (2001) introduced the idea of the 'heart health programme' to provide extended rehabilitation and provided information in a step-by-step process. The first two weeks focused on recovery and wound care, progressing to functional ability by week 3. The focus of the programme by 7–12 weeks was on returning to work, social activities and any lifestyle changes. This internet-based programme allowed health care staff to input individual profiles, monitor response and offer on line support.

Pulmonary rehabilitation

Whether or not a formal rehabilitation programme is appropriate for patients following thoracic surgery will depend on a number of factors, not least the diagnosis and surgical procedure performed. It is likely that only a small number of patients will enter a formal rehabilitation programme and careful selection is important. The focus in pulmonary rehabilitation is different from that on other programmes and involves assisting the patient reach maximal potential within the limits of their own disease and being able to live with a respiratory disability with improved quality of life (Rudkin 2001). Programmes might include some of the following components:

- Chest physiotherapy with the teaching of effective breathing exercises
- Improving general posture and fitness
- Pharmacological management
- Nutritional intake
- Occupational therapy (energy conservation and work simplification)
- Counselling and support

Pulmonary rehabilitation frequently includes some form of respiratory exercises combined with education and has been found to significantly improve exercise endurance and perception of dyspnoea in chronic lung disease. It is this patient group where most research has been carried out, but pulmonary rehabilitation may be suitable for some patients before and after lung resection, lung transplantation and volume reduction surgery (Singh 1997). Gentle exercise may increase confidence and sense of well-being even though there may be no objective improvement in pulmonary function. Chest wall pain as a result of surgery can lead to stiffness and be very debilitating, and benefits may be gained from postural awareness education and techniques involving muscle and ligament stretching (Phillips & Allanby 1998). Physical therapy may also help to prevent poor posture where there is a lateral thoracotomy incision. When exercising under supervised conditions, the patient may become less fearful of dyspnoea and this may be due to a degree of desensitisation. Using self-efficacy theory the strength of belief about one's ability influences outcome and may therefore form a useful basis for a modified pulmonary rehabilitation programme for patients following thoracic surgery.

Respiratory muscle training has been investigated for its effect when implemented as a part of pulmonary rehabilitation (Riera *et al.* 2001). By increasing muscle strength the sensation of respiratory effort will be reduced as will anxiety. There is limited evidence that respiratory muscle training alone will impact upon exercise capacity and quality of life and so should be just one facet of a comprehensive programme (Lacasse *et al.* 1997). Skills training such as breathing exercises, strategies to reduce dyspnoea and improve functional ability may assist with retraining and so reduce distress and anxiety associated with breathlessness. Health promotion is still an important area, and although the zeal with which risk modification teaching is taught may need to be tempered, guidance is still necessary on how to optimise health potential associated with activities of daily living.

Promoting patient confidence

An important factor determining success of all strategies previously explored is the relationship between patient and health provider. Hopefully, patients are no longer passive recipients of health care, but if self-management is to become more than rhetoric then health professionals need to look at how, often unintentionally, they may still be fostering a degree of paternalism.

Most developed countries are having to develop more effective health strategies to cope with the ever increasing numbers of chronically ill within their populations. In the UK the idea of the 'expert patient' was set out in the government's 1999 White Paper *Saving Lives: Our Healthier Nation* (DoH 1999). Self-management initiatives are seen as crucial where patients can become key decision makers in the treatment process. Self-management programmes can be specifically designed to reduce the severity of symptoms and improve confidence, resourcefulness and self-efficacy. Developments such as this have taken place over the past 20 years with growing recognition that patients with chronic disorders deal with common issues such as pain management, stress and a need to develop coping skills on a daily basis. Topics addressed in programmes, therefore, must include cognitive factors, symptom management, exercise, nutrition, problem solving and communication with professionals. An important aspect of these programmes is that there are trained lay people with chronic illness as tutors, and they can operate at a number of different levels:

- Hospital
- Primary care
- Patients' organisations
- Health and social care professionals

As we have explored in this chapter, patient self-management is not simply about educating patients about their condition: it also involves their developing the confidence and motivation to use their own skills, information and professional services to take effective control over life once discharged from formal health care.

In North America the increase in patients with chronic illness has led to the emergence, in primary care settings, of patient care teams in disease management (Wagner *et al.* 1997; Wagner 1998). Indeed, there is increasing international support for such an approach where similar problems have been encountered, including uncoordinated arrangements for delivering care, a bias towards acute treatment, a neglect of preventive care, and inappropriate treatment (Hunter 2000). Patient care teams may involve professionals outside the group of individuals working in a single practice, may involve multiple practices including primary and specialist care, or may involve multiple organisations, such as a general practice and a community agency (Wagner 2000). The effectiveness of this approach is often enhanced where nurses are involved in case management.

Figure 7.4 identifies possible support mechanisms for patients following surgery and highlights the many opportunities available for collaboration between all sectors and professionals. There is an assumption that budgets are pooled and primary, social and community services are under the same roof. Currently, however, although progress is being made in some areas, geographical, professional and philosophical divisions still need to be overcome for seamless care to become a reality.

Self-management, by addressing skills acquisition and cognitive and social determinants of behaviour, can improve patient motivation and confidence. Specialist nurses are ideally placed to play an active role, with success already demonstrated in patients following MI (DeBusk *et al.* 1994), and in elderly patients with congestive cardiac failure (Rich *et al.* 1995). Specialist nurses may be particularly effective in managing the complex needs of the cardiothoracic surgical patient in collaboration with other providers in the primary care setting. Prospective studies are needed to explore the home care needs and health patterns of cardiothoracic surgical patients in more depth, using standardised instruments to examine the relationships between function, cognition, psychosocial variables, symptoms and outcomes of home care (Redeker & Brassard 1996).

In the past decade great emphasis has been placed upon education and counselling as a part of rehabilitation, and as the period of hospitalisation has decreased, such education is increasingly undertaken on an outpatient basis. Improved knowledge about slowing disease progression has been translated to the patient through education. However, cognitive information alone is insufficient to bring about disease retardation and skills training or retraining and motivation are important components of this aftercare. New technologies, such as electronic databases and software, can also be utilised to enhance the delivery of

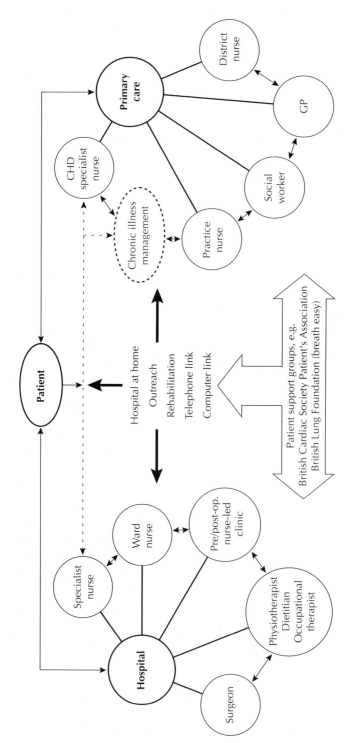

Fig. 7.4 Support mechanism and professional collaboration following discharge.

care to the person returning home after major cardiothoracic surgery. These technologies can facilitate the tracking of patients and the information they have received, can store data regarding the process of recovery and provide data for evaluation and audit. Additionally, they can be used to provide high quality instructions to the patient from a distance, tailored to their process of recovery.

Finally, health care providers need to be innovative in their approach in supporting patients once discharged. There are exciting possibilities for cardiothoracic surgical nurses, especially as traditional boundaries are being removed with real possibilities in the development of collaborative delivery models between primary and secondary sectors.

References

AACPR (American Association for Cardiovascular and Pulmonary Rehabilitation) (1999) *Guidelines for Cardiac Rehabilitation and Secondary Prevention Programmes*, 3rd edn. Human Kinetics, Illinois.

Ades, P., Waldman, M., McCann, W. & Weaver, S. (1992) Predictors of cardiac rehabilitation participation in older coronary patients. *Archives of Internal Medicine* **152**: 1033–5.

Ajzen, I. & Fishbein, M. (1980) *Understanding Attitudes and Predicting Behaviour.* Prentice Hall, Englewood Cliffs, NJ.

Amick, T.L. & Ockene, J.K. (1994) The role of social support in the modification of risk factors for cardiovascular disease. In: Shumaker, S.A. & Cajkowski, S.M. (eds) *Social Support and Cardiovascular Disease.* Plenum Press, New York.

Bandura, A. (1977) Self efficacy: toward a unifying theory of behavioural change. *Psychological Review* **84**: 191–215.

Bowles, K. & Danskey, K. (2001) Teaching self-management of diabetes via telehome care. *Home Health Care Nurse* **20**(1): 36–42.

Brennan, P., Moore, S., Bkornsdottir, G., Jones, J., Visovsky, C. & Rogers, M. (2001) Heartcare: an internet based information and support system for patient home recovery after coronary artery bypass grafting surgery. *Journal of Advanced Nursing* **35**(5): 699–708.

Carrel, T. & Mohacsi, P. (1998) Optimal timing of rehabilitation after cardiac surgery: the surgeon's view. *European Heart Journal* **19** (Supple. 0) 038–041.

Claxton, A., Cramer, J. & Pierce, C. (2001) A systematic review of the associations between dose regimen and medication compliance. *Clinical Therapeutics.* **23**(8): 1296–1310.

Cykert, S., Kissling, G. & Hansen, C.J. (2000) Patient preferences regarding outcomes after lung resection: what outcomes should preoperative evaluations target? *Chest* **117**: 1551–9.

DeBusk, R.F., Houston-Miller, N., Superko, R. *et al.* (1994) A case management system for coronary risk factor modification after acute myocardial infarction. *Annals of Internal Medicine* **120**: 721–9.

DoH (Department of Health) (1999) *Saving Lives: Our Healthier Nation.* The Stationery Office, London.

DoH (Department of Health) (2000)*The National Service Framework for Coronary Heart Disease.* The Stationery Office, London.

Dunstan, J. & Riddle, M. (1997) Rapid recovery management: the effects on the patient who has undergone heart surgery. *Heart and Lung* **26**(4): 289–98.

Handy, J.R., Asaph, J.W., Skokan, L. *et al.* (2002) What happens to patients undergoing lung cancer surgery? Outcomes and quality of life before and after surgery. *Chest* **122**(1): 21–30.

Harpham, W.S. (1999) Resolving the frustration of fatigue. *CA: A Cancer Journal for Clinicians* **49**: 178–89.

Helgeson, V.S. & Taylor, S.E. (1993) Social comparisons and adjustment among cardiac patients. *Journal of Applied Social Psychology* **3**: 1171–95.

Heller, R., Knapp, J., Valenti, L. & Dobson, A. (1993) Secondary prevention after acute myocardial infarction. *American Journal of Cardiology* 759–62.

Hunter, D.J. (2000) Disease management: has it a future? *British Medical Journal* **320**(7324): 530–31.

Jackson, G., Betteridge, J., Dean, J. *et al.* (1999) A systematic approach to erectile dysfunction in the cardiovascular patient: a consensus statement. *International Journal of Clinical Practice* **53**(6): 445–51.

Jaarsma, T., Kastermans, M., Dassen, T. & Philipsen, H. (1995) Problems of cardiac patients in early recovery. *Journal of Advanced Nursing* **21**(1): 21–7.

Jenkins, L.S. & Gortner, S.R. (1998) Correlates of self efficacy expectation and prediction of walking behaviour in cardiac surgery elders. *Annals of Behavioral Medicine* **20**(2): 99–103.

Jickling, J. & Graydon, J. (1997) The information needs at time of hospital discharge of male and female patients who have undergone coronary artery bypass grafting: a pilot study. *Heart and Lung* **26**: 350–57.

Johnson, K. (2000) Use of telephone follow-up for post cardiac surgery patients. *Intensive and Critical Care Nursing* **16**: 144–50.

Kerns, R. & Weiss, L. (1994) Family influences on the course of chronic illness: a cognitive-behavioural transaction. *Annals of Behavioural Medicine* **16**: 116–21.

Kulik, J.A., Mahler, H.I. & Moore, P.J. (1996) Social comparison and affiliation under threat: effects on recovery from major surgery. *Journal of Personality and Social Psychology* **71**: 967–79.

Lacasse, Y., Guyatt, G. & Goldstein, R. (1997) The components of a respiratory rehabilitation program: a systematic overview. *Chest* **111**(4): 1077–88.

Lazar, H., Fitzgerald, C., Ahmad, T. *et al.* (2001) Early discharge after coronary artery bypass surgery: are patients really going home earlier? *Journal of Thoracic and Cardiovascular Surgery* **121**(5): 943–50.

Maglish, B., Schwartz, J. & Matheny, R. (1999) Outcomes improvement following minimally invasive direct coronary artery bypass surgery. *Critical Care Nursing Clinics of North America* **11**(2): 177–88.

Mangione, C.N., Goldman, L., Orav, E.J. *et al.* (1997) Health related quality of life after elective surgery: measurement of longitudinal changes. *Journal of General Medicine* **12**: 686–97.

Margereson, C. (2001) Living with chronic respiratory illness and breathlessness. In: Esmond, G. (ed.) *Respiratory Nursing.* Baillière Tindall, Edinburgh.

Melville, M., Packham, C., Brown, N., Weston, C. & Gray, D. (1999) Cardiac rehabilitation: socially deprived patients are less likely to attend but patients ineligible for thrombolysis are less likely to be invited. *Heart* **82**(3): 373–7.

Moore, S. (1995) A comparison of women's and men's symptoms during home recovery after coronary artery bypass surgery. *Heart and Lung* **24**(6): 495–501.

Moore, S., Ruland, C., Pashkow, F. & Blackburn, G. (1998) Women's patterns of exercise following cardiac rehabilitation. *Nursing Research* **47**: 318–24.

Moser, D. (1994) Social support and cardiac recovery. *Journal of Cardiovascular Nursing* **9**(1): 27–36.

Muller, J., Mittleman, M., Maclure, M., Sherwood, J. & Tofler, G. (1996) Triggering myocardial infarction by sexual activity: low absolute risk and prevention by regular physical exertion. *Journal of American Medical Association* **275**(18): 1405–9.

Nakai, Y., Kataoka, Y., Bando, M. *et al.* (1987) Effects of physical exercise training on cardiac function and graft patency after coronary artery bypass grafting. *Journal of Thoracic Cardiovascular Surgery* **93**: 65–72.

Ng, J. & Tam, S. (2000) Effect of exercise based cardiac rehabilitation on mobility and self-esteem of persons after cardiac surgery. *Perceptual and Motor Skills* **91**(1): 107–14.

O'Connor, G., Buring, J., Yusef, S. *et al.* (1989) An overview of randomised trials of rehabilitation with exercise after myocardial infarction. *Circulation* **65**(Suppl. III): 115–19.

Oldridge, N., Ragowski, B. & Gottlieb, M. (1992) Use of outpatient cardiac rehabilitation services: factors associated with attendance. *Journal of Cardiopulmonary Rehabilitation* **12**: 25–31.

Penque, S., Petersen, B., Arom, K., Ratner, E. & Halm, M. (1999) Early discharge with home health care I: the coronary artery bypass patient. *Dimensions of Critical Care Nursing* **18**(6): 40–48.

Phillips, G. & Allanby, C. (1998) Pulmonary rehabilitation in chronic respiratory insufficiency. In: Shuldham, C. (ed.) *Cardiorespiratory Nursing*. Stanley Thornes, Cheltenham.

Prochaska, J.O. & DiClemente, C.C. (1984) *The Transtheoretical Approach: Crossing Traditional Foundations of Change*. Dow Jones/Irwin, Homewood, IL.

Redeker, N.S. & Brassard, A.B. (1996) Health patterns of cardiac surgery clients using home health care nursing services. *Public Health Nursing* **13**(6): 394–403.

Rich, M.W., Beckham, V., Wittenberg, C., Leven, C.L., Freedland, K.E. & Carney, R.M. (1995) A multidisciplinary intervention to prevent the readmission of elderly patients with congestive cardiac failure. *New England Journal of Medicine* **333**: 1130–95.

Riegal, B. (1989) Social support and psychological adjustment to chronic coronary heart disease: operationalisation in Johnson's behavioural systems model. *Advances in Nursing Science* **11**: 74–84.

Riegal, B., Gates, D., Gocka, I. *et al.* (1996) Effectiveness of a program of early hospital discharge of cardiac surgery patients. *Journal of Cardiovascular Nursing* **11**(1): 63–75.

Riera, H., Rubio, T., Ruiz, F. *et al.* (2001) Inspiratory muscle training in patients with COPD. *Chest* **120**(3): 748–56.

Roebuck, A. (1999) Telephone support in the early discharge period following elective cardiac surgery: does it reduce anxiety and depression levels? *Intensive and Critical Care Nursing* **15**: 142–6.

Ross, A., Brodie, E., Carroll, D., Nivens, C. & Hotchkiss, R. (2000) The psychosocial and physical impact of exercise rehabilitation following coronary artery bypass surgery. *Coronary Health Care* **4**: 63–70.

Rudkin, S. (2001) Pulmonary rehabilitation. In: Esmond, G. (ed.) *Respiratory Nursing*. Baillière Tindall, Edinburgh.

Sharma, R. & McLeod, A. (2001) Cardiac rehabilitation after coronary artery bypass graft surgery: its effect on ischaemia, functional capacity, and a multivariate index of prognosis. *Coronary Health Care* **5**: 189–93.

Singh, S.J. (1997) Patient selection and assessment for pulmonary rehabilitation. In: Morgan, M. & Singh, S. (eds) *Practical Pulmonary Rehabilitation*. Chapman & Hall, London.

Skarvan, K. (2000) Ventricular performance. In: Priebe, H. & Skevan, K. (eds) *Cardiovascular Physiology*, 2nd edn. BMJ Publishing Group, London.

Smith, J. & Kampine, J. (1990) *Circulatory Physiology – The Essentials*, 3rd edn. Williams & Wilkins, Baltimore.

Speziale, G., Ruvolo, G. & Marino, B. (1996) Quality of life following coronary bypass surgery. *Journal of Cardiovascular Surgery* **37**: 75–8.

Stricklin, M., Jones, S. & Niles, S. (2000) Home talk/health talk: improving patients' health status with telephone technology. *Home Healthcare Nurse* **18**(1): 53–61.

Tardif, G. (1989) Sexual activity after a myocardial infarction. *Archives of Medical Rehabilitation* **70**: 763–6.

Thomas, R., Millen, N., Lanendola, C. *et al.* (1996) National survey on gender differences in cardiac rehabilitation programmes: patient characteristics and enrolment patterns. *Journal of Cardiopulmonary Rehabilitation* **16**: 402–12.

Thompson, D. & Lewin, R. (2000) Management of the post-myocardial infarction patient: rehabilitation and cardiac neurosis. *Heart* **84**(1): 101–5.

Thompson, D., Bowman, G., Kitson, A., deBono, D. & Hopkins, A. (1996) Cardiac rehabilitation in the United Kingdom: guidelines and audit standards. *Heart* **75**: 89–93.

Tilden, V. & Weinert, C. (1987) Social support and the chronically ill individual. *Nursing Clinics of North America* **22**: 613–20.

Wagner, E.H. (1998) Chronic disease management: what will it take to improve care for chronic illness? *Effective Clinical Practice* **1**(1): 2–4.

Wagner, E.H. (2000) The role of patient care teams in chronic disease management. *British Medical Journal* **320**(7234): 569–72.

Wagner, E.H., Davis, C., Schaaefer, J., Von Korff, M. & Austin, B. (1997) A survey of leading chronic disease management programmes: are they consistent with the literature? *Managed Care Quarterly* **3**: 56–66.

Wright, D., Williams, S., Riley, R., Marshall, P. & Tan, L. (2002) Is early, low level, short term exercise cardiac rehabilitation following coronary bypass surgery beneficial? A randomised controlled trial. *Heart* **88**: 83–4.

Yerge-Cole, G. (2001) On the alert for pregnancy induced hypertension. *Home Healthcare Nursing* **19**(11): 727–8.

Yun, K.L., Sintek, C.F., Fletcher, A.D. *et al.* (1999) Time related quality of life after elective cardiac operation. *Annals of Thoracic Surgery* **68**: 1314–20.

Further reading

Department of Health (2002) *The Expert Patient: A New Approach to Chronic Disease Management for the 21st Century*. The Stationery Office, London.

Wyer, S., Earl, L., Joseph, S. & Harrison, J. (2001) Deciding whether to attend a cardiac rehabilitation programme: an interpretive phenomenological analysis. *Coronary Health Care* **5**(4): 178–88.

Index